INTEGRATIVE NUTRITION

THE FUTURE OF NUTRITION

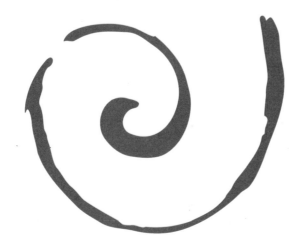

BY JOSHUA ROSENTHAL

acknowledgments

Along the path of life, God and the universe guide us to interact with certain people. The following individuals have significantly contributed to who I am today and how I am today, and I thank them for all our interactions.

My dear parents for their unconditional love and support • My brother Yaakov and his family • My many uncles, aunts and cousins • Nathan Patmor, the driving force at Integrative Nutrition over the past few years • Shirley Thompson, dedicated to the long-term vision of the school • Abina Benson whose brilliance and support are always present • Tricia Napor, the main person who helped bring this book to life • Nancy Wagner • Dr. Laytner • Norman Shaul • Tommy Hoffstedter • Alice Grosz • David Rosensweig • Norman Weisbart • Benjie Applebaum • Jacob Buksbaum • Larry Shemen • Sambo • Dave and Jimmy Diamond • Bill House • Allan Gould • Dave Mann • Cat Stevens • Chaim Friedman • Azriel Haimowitz • Devorah Kahn • Meyer Weiss • Gary Gershoni • Nick Hannah • Hellen Klyle • Dr. Klein • Joel Sadavoy • Leslie Ungar • George Hanson • Mr. Mackenzie • Aimee Gagné • Christine Sutherland • Grace Chan • Irene van DeLagemaat • Karen Ball • Mary Bottomley • Sheron Tyminski • Malca Narrol • Michio and Aveline Kushi • Carolyn Heidendry • Diane Silver • Chris Hassel • Anne Marie Colbin • Sanja Nikolic • Arlindo • Chris Sartor • Val • Kathy Walker • Patty Rehmer • Pendra • Jeannie Butler • Dean Ornish • Sherri Rogers • Blake Gould • Murray Snyder • Bill and Joanie Spear • Verne Varona • Shizuko Yamamoto • Takashi Yoshikawa • Lino and Jane Stanchich • Bill Tara • Sandy Pukel • Werner Erhardt • Justin Sterling • Martin Rutte • Robert Panté • Amrit Desai • Stephen Shannon • Nick Ashfield • Tony Robbins • Paulo Coelho • Osho • Anando • Yogendra • Margot Anand • Kosha • Sohini • Dolano • Ganga-ji • Byron Katie • Anudas • Bahulya • Sagar • Shikha • Salina • Francina • Omega • Silvaraj • Lily • Subhuti • Picky • Giri • Manoj • Rita • Shira • Thaysha • Ma Faiza • Meera • Ranie • Ganga • Bhakti • Dr. Phulphagar • Marcie and Michael Zaroff • Surya • Patricia James • Jessica Porter • Carolina de Bartolo • Betsy Esser • Allison Jobson • Liat Solomon • Alok Zemach • Darshana Weill • Jennette Turner • Carin McKay • Steve and Ashley Bearman • Jenn Breckenridge • Adley Gartenstein • Jasmine Aucott • Alice Moore • Tysan Lerner • Jason Brown • Robyn Holt • Robin Peglow • Fabienne Fredrickson • Karin Witzig • Deb Fischman • Doris Ingber • Lisa Wrona • Craig Hazen • Patricia Grimsley • Shaly Sharma • Krisztina Szilvasi • Elishia Trotter • Jessie Caven • Rhian Watson • Liyana Silver • Leigh van Swall • Christine Whitmire • Chelsea Polak • Winnie Jamieson • Teri Myers • Connie Chan • Christine Meyers • Katherine Constable • Joanna Palazzolo • Katie Zeiner • Jessica Cary • Brian Long • Jesika Brenna • Lyle Beers • Freddy Rodrigues • Julie Averill • Benjamin Leavitt • Sara Norman • Brooke Schechtman • Jess Rude • Laura Martin • Theresa Palazzo • Jen Ward • Juliet Smith • Wilma Medina • Meredith Ian • Rose Payne • Sigi Weiss • Leda Dederich • Rusty Ross • James Coleman • Rachel Fireman • Jean Marie Truchard • Allison Carmen • Elie El Saddick • Michael Hiller • Howard Schain • Gary Krauthamer • Marc and Meryl Rudin • Stephan Rechtschaffen • Annette • Thierry • Walter Beebee • Gabrielle Roth • Julia Cameron • Julia Butterfly Hill • Deepak Chopra • Queen Afua • Neal Barnard • Andrea Beaman • James D'Adamo • Marc David • John Douillard • Sally Fallon • Steve Gagné • Oz Garcia • Cara Hogue • Colette Heimowitz • Joseph Mercola • Tom Monte • Marion Nestle • Christianne Northrup • Paul Pitchford • Barry Sears • Andrew Weil • Walter Willet • David Wolfe • Victor Zeines • Master Herbert • Petrina Plecko • Liat Solomon • Rebecca Menashe • Grace Hickey • Cory Thompson • Christine Waltermyer • Tom • Lora Dibner • Ty Geysuk • Holly Shelowitz • Susan Rubin • Santha Cooke • Linsey Francesca Paik • Dan Topkis • Dawn Davis • Teresa Hurst • Juliette Closset • Stephen Pollitt • Jena la Flamme • Sundarah Eubanks • Aarona Pichinson • Maria DiSalvo • Maria Gamb • Dara Kessler • Molly Lee • Alisa Vitti • Dorothy Kozlowski • Shashi Martynova • Riikka Rajamaki • Tamara Xavier • Kristin Blozie • Rebecca Feldman • Andrea Wulwick • Marcie Goldman • Kristen Frost • Miriam Adler • Donna Terjesen • Lucia Luna • Pam Rich • Veronica Ortiz • Pauline Perez • Teresa Kay-Aba Kennedy • Mayumi Nishimura • Eri Shigaguchi • Rajanila Kubota • Dharma • Yumi • Lilla • Michiko • Anna Chisholm • Sandy Chasteen • Shelley Lepage • Melissa King • Meryem Kabsy • Afya Ibomu • Fiona Chan • Christi Lehner • Alex Jamieson • Katherine Jamieson • Cynthia Stadd • Margot Schulman • Deborah Dunn • Allison Goldschlag • Susan Banzon • James Chew • Leesaw Andaloro • Debra Duby • Caryn Fishlevich • Lisa Graham • Lisa Jacobson • Carolynn Kent • Christina May • Robert Notter • Jeanne Reilly • Kerri Roberts • Nike Steinberg • Liselle Swanson • Karen Morales • Tina Yakuwa • Farah Gokturk • Francesca Leone • Mario Hewitt • Reid Mihalko • Laura Melillo • Mount Allen • Pat Napor • Jennifer Moore • Erika Tsoukanelis • Laura Ogar

All the clients, students, immersionists and alumni who have attended the school, anyone who ever purchased my books, joined the school's mailing list, and basically everyone I've ever met. You've all helped to get me where I am today. With all my heart, thank you!

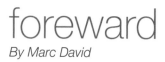

foreward

By Marc David

H AVE YOU NOTICED THAT AN EXTRA large portion of our collective conversation around nutrition is driven by our love for the exaggerated excitement of "what's new"—the latest, miraculous supplement for limitless energy, the hottest diet that guarantees fat free glamour, or the next breakthrough food that defies disease and attracts your perfect mate? We expect quite a bit from food, and perhaps rightly so. But is there really anything new worth getting excited over? Are any of the breakthrough pills, foods or gizmos truly delivering on their promises? If we gaze honestly and compassionately at the illness, obesity and unhappiness surrounding us, the answer appears to be a poignant "no." We've looked to the science of nutrition to lead us into the promised land of milk and honey, but upon arrival we've been told "don't drink the milk" and "don't eat the honey." And to make things more confusing for eaters everywhere, our nutrition experts are ceaselessly engaged in a war over who holds the key to the kingdom called "The Right Way to Eat."

Fortunately, things are changing. There really is something new in nutrition, and it's this: a holistic understanding of food and health that embraces all of who we are as eaters—body, mind, heart, soul, spirit and planet. This broader vision affirms that each of us is biochemically unique, that there's no "one size fits all" in the diet business, and that every nutritional system or expert has at least one nugget of wisdom to offer us.

The Institute for Integrative Nutrition is the nesting ground for this new paradigm of nutritional health. It's the power spot where a fresh vision of our relationship with food is being birthed into practical, real-world manifestation. The Institute has filled a huge void with resounding success. The results are seen in the great number of students and graduates who are inspired about their work and fueled by the inner knowing that they are nutritional innovators sharing a special gift with the world.

I love teaching at Integrative Nutrition because the students are world-class. They're there to learn, ready to grow, eager to share, and willing to step into a vast new territory in nutritional health. The diversity of the student body adds to the charm of the Institute, and the life experience each student brings to the classroom enriches and inspires. Of course, the staff is solidly committed to delivering an education grounded in excellence, and they create a beautiful container for deep learning to naturally take place. I'm honored to be a part of this special experience.

It's also a pleasure for me to watch the intellectual and personal unfoldment that students experience at Integrative Nutrition. They have a sense of aliveness that's rare and refreshing. Indeed, students continually face head-on the greatest challenge in the field of nutrition today—the severe, long-term deficiency of vitamin L—love, and vitamin S—soul. They intuitively recognize that we are more than just a collection of chemicals, and food is more than the sum total of its vitamins, minerals and macronutrients.

For too many years, the psychological and spiritual dimensions of eating have been banished from the table. As a result, we've suffered from simplistic and ineffective nutritional strategies such as "eat less and exercise more" or "eat this, don't eat that." We've given our power away to outside authorities, to punishing forms of diet and fitness, and to impossible standards of health and beauty. The Institute for Integrative Nutrition is a rare haven of relief from this outdated approach, and a nourishing force in health education unlike any other.

As someone interested in nutrition and well-being, you've chosen a special way to nourish yourself. Congratulations. It's now your task to liberate yourself from the kind of negative inner dialogue where you judge your own health, weight, and way of eating and living in the world. In the process, you'll learn how to help others. Remember to honor your inner knowing. Respect your gift. Stop feeding your imperfections so much time and energy. You don't need to be perfect, fit, beautiful, and in luminous emotional and medical health to help people. Your task is not to learn to fix anyone. Just be real, be honest, be compassionate and be you. Accept where you are with graceful, loving courage, and your success is ensured. Your gift to the nutrition world is your own journey in all its fullness. Go out and share it as if it were the best meal on Earth.

Marc David
Boulder, Colorado
Author of *The Slow Down Diet and Nourishing Wisdom*

table of contents

Introduction *ix*

How to Use This Book *xi*

Chapter 1 Question What You're Told *1*

The USDA Food Guide Pyramid • Politics of Food • Food Corporations • Contemporary Eating Habits

• The New Dietary Guidelines • MyPyramid • Government Policy • Supersized Nation • Just Say No to Drugs

• The American Dietetic Association • The Turning Point

EXERCISES *15* Supermarket Field Trip • Examine MyPyramid • Watch *Supersize Me* • Trustworthy Professionals

GRADUATE PROFILE *17* Devon's story

Chapter 2 Foundations of Integrative Nutrition *19*

Bio-Individuality • The Laboratory of Your Body • The Lost Art of Listening • Food-Mood Journal

• Energy of Food • Food Quality • Metabolic Rate • Hunger and Binging • Crowding Out • When We Eat

• How We Eat • The Importance of Chewing • Explore Your Body

EXERCISES *32* The Breakfast Experiment • Metabolic Type Test • Mindful Eating GRADUATE PROFILE *35* Teresa's story

Chapter 3 Dietary Theory *37*

Macrobiotics • Ayurveda • 5 Element Theory • High Carbohydrate Diets • High Protein Diets

• The Zone Diet • South Beach Diet • Blood Type Diet • Sally Fallon Diet • Raw Food Diet

• Master Cleanser • Joshua's 90-10 Diet • Finding the Right Diet for You

EXERCISE *58* Creating Your Own Diet GRADUATE PROFILE *59* Julia's story

Chapter 4 Deconstructing Cravings *61*

Sugar-Addicted Client • Simple and Complex Carbohydrates • Kevin's Story • Food Our Ancestors Ate •

• Now, My Ice Cream Story • Cravings Are Not a Problem • Contracting and Expanding Foods • Crazy Cravings

• Your Body Loves You

EXERCISES *74* Craving Inventory • Tongue Scraper • Dearest Body of Mine GRADUATE PROFILE *77* Robert's story

Chapter 5 Primary Food *79*

Relationships • Career • Physical Activity • Spirituality • Our Food Pyramid

EXERCISE *90* The Circle of Life GRADUATE PROFILE *91* Rose's story

Chapter 6 Escape the Matrix *93*

The Matrix • Hungry? Why Wait? • The Pressure to Be Thin • Superwoman Syndrome • Superman Syndrome • The Individual • Fitting Out

EXERCISES *102* Turn Off the Media • Wish List • Hot Water Bottle GRADUATE PROFILE *105* Alisa's story

Chapter 7 The Integrative Nutrition Plan: 12 Steps to Health *107*

Drink More Water • Practice Cooking • Increase Whole Grains • Increase Sweet Vegetables • Increase Leafy Green Vegetables • Experiment with Protein • Less Meat, Dairy, Sugar, Chemicalized Artificial Junk Foods; Less Coffee, Alcohol and Tobacco • Develop Easy and Reliable Ways to Nurture Your Body • Have Healthy Relationships That Support You • Find Physical Activity You Enjoy and Do It Regularly • Find Work You Love Or a Way to Love the Work You Have • Develop a Spiritual Practice

EXERCISES *120* Your First Step • Hot Towel Scrub GRADUATE PROFILE *121* Donna's story

Chapter 8 Foods to Avoid or Minimize *123*

Sugar • Dairy • Meat • Coffee • Salt • Chocolate

EXERCISES *133* Reduce One Food • Be Bad GRADUATE PROFILE *135* Steve's story

Chapter 9 Cooking Like Your Life Depends On It *137*

Homemade • Freshly Made • Lovingly Made • Simplicity • Use a Timer • Burn the Rice • Add Flavor • Cook Once, Eat Two or Three Times • Notice the Effects of Your Cooking • Cooking with the Seasons • Restaurant Eating • Flexitarian

EXERCISES *146* Condiment List • Try a New Recipe GRADUATE PROFILE *147* Dianna's story

Chapter 10 Why Be Healthy? *149*

Authentic Self-Expression • Unpredictable Futures • Spiritual Beings • Building Your Future

EXERCISE *154* Future-Building Exercise GRADUATE PROFILE *157* Debbie's story

Recipes *159*

Simple Grains *161* • Vegetables *168* • Beans *176* • Tofu and Tempeh *182* • Meat and Fish *186* • Soups *190* • Salads *194* • Salad Dressings *199* • Sea Vegetables *200* • Savory Snacks *202* • Desserts *208* • Your Basic Shopping List *212*

GRADUATE PROFILE *214* Jena's story

Epilogue *217*

Book References *219*

introduction

AMERICA IS A GREAT COUNTRY. WE HAVE
the security, freedom and lifestyle desired by many people around the world. But Americans are overweight,
unhappy and unhealthy. Every year healthcare costs increase while overall health decreases; people continue
to eat poorly, gain weight and depend on medications and operations to maintain their health.

We can do better. Americans deserve an effective, efficient system based on prevention, holistic health
education, sound nutrition theory and high quality personal care. Integrative Nutrition is dedicated to
helping evolve the future of nutrition, so that all beings can live healthier, happier, more fulfilling lives. We
are called the Institute for Integrative Nutrition because we teach a way of eating that synthesizes the best
of all the different nutrition theories, from the ancient traditions of Ayurveda, macrobiotics and Chinese
medicine to the most current concepts like raw foods, Atkins, the Blood Type Diet, the Zone and the
USDA Pyramid. There is no perfect way of eating that works for everyone. We believe in intuitive eating,
based on the idea that what's right for one person may not be right for another.

As more Americans adopt a healthier lifestyle, this great country will strengthen itself from the inside
out and become a model for others around the world. We are looking to you to be an important part of
this transformation. As our health improves, we feel empowered to pursue the life of our dreams —the
life we came here to live. Our intention is for you to uncover this process for yourself and then share
it with others. The public wants to be healthy. They are thrilled to have teachers and counselors with a
broad understanding of health and nutrition to show them the way.

If this book found its way to you or you found your way to this book, we trust it means you are a
highly intelligent, highly sensitive human being with an appreciation for the benefits of whole foods and
holistic living. Our mission is to empower you to stand up, speak up and act up for what you believe to
be true. You are a brilliant individual with the capacity to reach out and touch many lives.

The faculty, staff, students and alumni at Integrative Nutrition wish you a wonderful life. May this
book assist you along the path towards a healthy, happy future for yourself, your family and your friends.
May your aliveness create a ripple effect in the world, and may all your hopes and dreams come true.

Until one is committed,
there is hesitancy,
the chance to draw back,
always ineffectiveness.

Concerning all acts
of initiative and creation,
there is one elementary truth
the ignorance of which
kills countless ideas and splendid plans:
that the moment one definitely commits oneself,
then providence moves too.

All sorts of things occur
to help one that would never
otherwise have occurred.
A whole stream of events
issues from the decision,
raising in one's favor all manner
of unforeseen incidents,
meetings and material assistance
which no man could have dreamed
would have come his way.

Whatever you can do
or dream you can, begin it.
Boldness has genius,
power and magic in it.
Begin it now.

Johann Wolfgang von Goethe

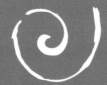

how to use this book

Intention The intention of this book is to permanently change your relationship to food and health. You will notice that when this happens, everything in your life will change. You will have a positive impact on the people around you. You may help them to change too, and when the people around you change, the world can change.

Discovery A permanent shift in health may seem like a big challenge requiring a lot of dedication, but this approach is not about acquiring more self-discipline or willpower. It's about personally discovering what nourishes you, what feeds you and what ultimately makes your life extraordinary. If you do not enjoy eating, you will not enjoy life. It's that simple.

Solving "the Problem" Many people feel that health and nutrition are serious issues. They are. But this doesn't mean you have to solve "the problem" of taking care of your body. You can change your diet and your life while having a good time.

Focus Devoting a small amount of time now to your personal nutrition will result in a different future later. I encourage you to read this book like your life depends on it because it does.

The Right Diet In this book, you will find discussion of major dietary theories. But the food that is best for you is not going to be found in the pages of a nutrition book. This book will help you reunite with your body's wisdom so you can easily make food choices that are appropriate for your unique body and lifestyle.

Do the Exercises The exercises contained in the following chapters have been carefully chosen to help you understand the dynamics of nutrition. If you come to understand how food affects you and how to eat, you will develop an entirely different outlook on life.

Make a Friendly Mess of This Book As you read, pick up a pen or highlighter and start underlining statements in these pages that feel especially important for you. You are invited to write all over this book. Take notes in the margins. Make it your own. Personalize it. Feel comfortable picking it up and putting it down. It's a workbook and a play book.

One Rung of the Ladder at a Time In this book you will unlearn old habits and absorb new information. Give yourself permission to go slowly. Big changes do not require big leaps. As far as your body is concerned, permanent change is more likely to happen gradually. Proceed with care for yourself. Have fun.

chapter 1

The doctor of the future
will give no medicine,
but will interest his patient
in the care of the human frame,
in diet and in the cause and
prevention of disease.
Thomas Edison

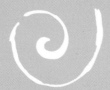

question what you're told

WHY ARE AMERICANS SO UNHEALTHY and overweight? Why are we suffering from increasing numbers of chronic health concerns, such as obesity, diabetes, reproductive issues and depression? Why do we need so much medical attention and medication? The answer to these questions lies in the fact that medicine has become a profit-driven industry. Medicine was originally established to be a source of health and healing, but the American government has a pro-business model instead of a pro-health model. They want to increase profit, decrease expenses and let the chips fall where they may. Wouldn't it be better to spend our money not on more pills and doctors bills, but on answering the question, What would it take to have a country full of healthy, happy people?

Our healthcare system is failing us. We pay increasingly more for health insurance, only to see our doctors less and get more prescriptions for medications. Health insurance today is really just pre-paid medical expenses. Paying our monthly fee does not promise health; it just ensures that if we get sick we won't have to pay in full for our medication or operation. What kind of system is this? According to a recent study by the World Health Organization, Americans spend far more, per capita, on healthcare than any other country, but somehow we rank only 37 in the world in terms of performance. How is this possible? If you went shopping in a store and were treated by a salesperson the way most health professionals treat their patients, chances are you would not go back to that store. For some reason, however, we continue to tolerate this archaic form of healthcare.

On top of skyrocketing prices for insurance and prescriptions, there is a growing gap between doctors and patients. The average doctor's visit is now three minutes. Patients want to know more about nutrition, supplements and prevention, while doctors are increasingly afraid of being sued and unhappy about being controlled by HMOs. It is predicted that by 2020 the U.S. will have a shortage of 100,000 physicians. America may have to start outsourcing and importing our doctors.

Before there were blood pressure units and stethoscopes, doctors in Asia went from village to village caring for their patients. Using their ancient, traditional and so-called primitive skills of diagnosis, they would ask a few questions, look into the patient's eyes, check their tongue, take their pulses and then make some recommendations. The next year, when the doctor returned, he was paid only if health was maintained. If there had been illness, the doctor was not paid. Now that's a good healthcare system!

I hope that the American public will become vocal about the high cost of healthcare and start questioning why they are paying so much money for drugs with dangerous side effects. Every year 2 million Americans become seriously ill due to toxic reactions to incorrectly prescribed medicines. Hello—where is the FDA? They are too focused on helping the drug companies maximize profit to actually think about what is best for the consumers. No one is saying, "Hey, maybe people don't need more drugs. Maybe they need to understand disease prevention, the importance of exercise and how to eat a healthy, balanced diet."

1991 USDA Food Guide Pyramid

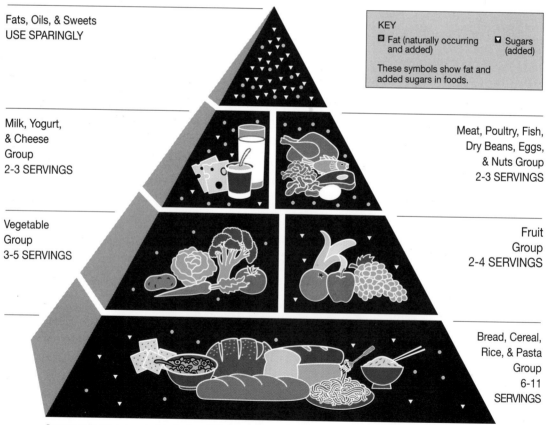

Fats, Oils, & Sweets
USE SPARINGLY

KEY
◻ Fat (naturally occurring and added)   ☑ Sugars (added)
These symbols show fat and added sugars in foods.

Milk, Yogurt, & Cheese Group
2-3 SERVINGS

Meat, Poultry, Fish, Dry Beans, Eggs, & Nuts Group
2-3 SERVINGS

Vegetable Group
3-5 SERVINGS

Fruit Group
2-4 SERVINGS

Bread, Cereal, Rice, & Pasta Group
6-11 SERVINGS

Source: U.S. Department of Agriculture/U.S. Department of Health and Human Services

Americans need to recognize the fundamental relationship between poor nutrition, expensive health-care and the lamentable state of the public's health. What we eat makes a huge difference in our health, yet very few doctors are educated about food—even the holistic ones. The more we are aware of our food and our body's messages, the less we have to depend on doctors and medication.

I founded the Institute for Integrative Nutrition to educate people about exactly these issues. Through our work, the work of our visiting faculty, our alumni and others in this community, we are creating a ripple effect that will transform the system into one that supports health and healing in all individuals.

• • • The USDA Food Guide Pyramid • • •

In 1991 the U.S. Department of Agriculture and the Department of Health and Human Services created the Food Guide Pyramid with the intended purpose of providing the public correct information about what to eat in order to be healthy. The medical profession, registered dietitians, insurance companies, politicians and bureaucrats all advocated this Food Guide Pyramid for 13 years.

To be accurate, the very first pyramid was never released. The meat and dairy industries blocked publication of the original pyramid because they claimed it stigmatized their products. Marion Nestle, professor and chair of the Department of Nutrition at New York University and guest lecturer at our institute, chronicled the saga in her pioneering book *Food Politics: How the Food Industry Influences Nutrition and Health*. According to Professor Nestle, the meat and dairy industries were upset because the first Food Guide Pyramid placed their products in a category labeled "eat less." The USDA then withdrew the guide and spent a lot of time and money trying to come up with a formula that would satisfy the two industries, and that's how the second, politically correct Food Guide Pyramid was created.

The federal dietary guidelines are reviewed every five years and updated if necessary, based on the latest scientific discoveries in nutrition. But since its first appearance in 1991, the Food Guide Pyramid stood more or less unchanged until April of 2005. Before looking at the latest changes, however, let's look at the original. The USDA used this pyramid to indicate the priority and quantity of each food group. As you can see, there are six food groups. The broad foundation is carbohydrates, including bread, cereal, rice and pasta. Next is a slightly narrower band of fruits and vegetables, then a smaller layer of protein-rich foods like meat and dairy. At the very top is a small section of fats, oils and sweets. Each of the six sections has a recommended number of servings, except the top section of fats, oils and sweets, which is accompanied by the advice "use sparingly."

This "use sparingly" in no way reflects what people actually eat. The fat in red meat, cheese and ice cream; the sugar in soft drinks, cookies and breakfast cereals; and the oil that seeped into the burger and fries at the fast food restaurant all add up to a daily intake that no definition of the word "sparingly'" can ever encompass.

The creators of the Food Guide Pyramid may protest that they had no control over what the public actually consumes, that their responsibilities ended with making the recommendations. The truth is, these recommendations were the very foundation of American attitudes about health, diet and nutrition. Over the past 13 years, Americans have experienced tremendous weight gain, deteriorating health and confusion about proper nutrition. This is largely due to the inaccuracies, deception and ambiguous information present in the Food Guide Pyramid.

Pressure on the government to appease the food industry is exercised primarily through Congress. Any senator or representative from Texas is going to support the red meat industry or he will not obtain campaign funds or votes to be re-elected. The same goes for politicians from dairy states like Wisconsin. These politicians are the people who, together with skilled, well-paid lobbyists, control legislation and information about nutrition put out by the government. Good nutrition is straightforward and simple, but in America today, food industry pressure makes it almost impossible for any public official to state the plain truth.

The government's uncomfortable position, torn between trying to protect the public on one hand and appease the food industry on the other, did not begin in 1991 with the creation of the pyramid. Back in 1977, the U.S. Senate Select Committee on Nutrition and Human Needs published its groundbreaking Dietary Goals for the U.S., which was the first government report to clearly show that excessive consumption of red meat, dairy products, eggs and processed foods was causing obesity and many serious illnesses. As a sensible and natural consequence, the original report contained a phrase advising Americans to decrease their consumption of red meat, but this was deleted under fierce pressure from the National Cattlemen's Beef Association. A similar situation continues today. In spite of heroic work by people like Professor Nestle, few Americans understand the extent to which public nutrition policy is dictated by the political process, which in turn is dictated by the corporate agenda to maximize profits.

• • • Food Corporations • • •

Food corporations are more or less free to deceive the public about the nature of their products, even using the Food Guide Pyramid as a vehicle for their own agenda. Advertisements created by Frito-Lay, the potato chip manufacturer, show several packets of chips with happy, smiling faces filling the bottom sectionof the USDA Food Guide Pyramid, implying that chips provide the carbohydrates you need for good health. This is nonsense. The carbohydrates in chips are so highly refined that, when consumed, they immediately break down into sugar in your body. They are also covered in fat and drenched in artificial flavoring.

Similarly, a widely distributed, brand name "health drink" boasts a label reading, "Complete, balanced nutrition to help stay healthy, active and energetic," plus the added claim, "No. 1 Doctor-recommended." On analysis, the drink contains four types of synthetic sweetener and some added vitamins. It is, in actuality, hyped-up sugar water. The supermarket shelf is a free-for-all in which anyone can claim almost anything, and public health authorities rarely interfere.

And it is not only in our country. People around the world are hungry for American products—movies, television shows, American cigarettes, and now American food. Convenience foods and fast food restaurants are sprouting up worldwide, and as our eating habits become fashionable in an increasing number of countries, so are our health concerns, such as obesity, diabetes and heart disease. The European Union is currently dealing with increasing obesity among children and adults, with experts predicting the figures will double over the next 20 years. On a recent trip to Japan, I was shocked at how much people's health has changed since I was there last, 12 years ago. At that time, the majority of people ate the traditional Japanese diet. Their bodies were slim, their skin was clear and there was a sense of tranquility everywhere. I was dismayed to see the increase in fast food restaurants, along with increased weight, skin conditions and stress among the people.

• • • Contemporary Eating Habits • • •

The important thing to understand is the way we are eating is new. Beginning at the turn of the 20th century and accelerating through to the present day, humans have replaced locally grown, home-cooked foods with processed, refined foods in which most of the nutrition is stripped away and chemicals are added to enhance flavor and sweetness. We have virtually stopped cooking, but are eating more than ever before.

What we buy in the store may be called food, may look like food, may taste like food, but it is not the food our great-grandmothers used to eat. When buying bread in the supermarket, we are actually buying a pre-packaged, pre-sliced loaf that is made from heavily refined white flour with additives that allow the bread to sit on the shelf for an extended period of time. When buying frozen fish filets, we are really buying pre-flavored fish with a brown, crispy shell that contains all kinds of chemicals.

Food isn't always as natural and wholesome as it looks. When we pop into the local fast food restaurant for a quick bite of deep-fried chicken, we're most likely getting something that was reared on a factory farm and fed a cocktail of hormones to make it grow quickly, weigh more, look good and taste right. If we buy a steak at the supermarket or a restaurant, chances are the animal was injected with a big dose of antibiotics just before traveling in a rail car to the slaughterhouse. This is a common practice to make sure cows don't get sick on the journey and deprive their owners of a well-earned buck. And it is not the first time the animal was given antibiotics. Cows are meant to eat grass, but because it is cheaper most are fed grains that cause bacteria to grow in their stomachs, so they are in need of antibiotics throughout their lifetimes. When we eat that steak, all those antibiotics end up in our bloodstream.

Gross meat info.

Sooner or later the effects of our contemporary eating habits have to become visible to the American public, in more ways than the increasing size of our waistlines.

• • • The New Dietary Guidelines • • •

Recent statistics forced the federal government to address the obesity issue, and this is why the guidelines were revised in an attempt to get Americans more healthy and fit. The USDA and the U.S. Department of Health and Human Services (HHS) released the latest Dietary Guidelines report in early 2005. It is described by its creators as "the most health-oriented ever," as it recommends Americans eat more vegetables and more whole grains, while cutting down on certain fats and consuming less sugar. The report also strongly recommends people "engage in regular physical activity and reduce sedentary activities to promote health, psychological well-being, and a healthy body weight." In other words: Get off your butt, America, and start exercising.

Tommy Thompson, HHS Secretary, announced:

These new Dietary Guidelines represent our best science-based advice to help Americans live healthier and longer lives. The report gives action steps to reach achievable goals in weight control, stronger muscles and bones, and balanced nutrition to help prevent chronic diseases such as heart disease, diabetes and some cancers. The process we used to develop these recommendations was more rigorous and more transparent than ever before. Taken together, the recommendations will help consumers make smart choices from every food group, get the most nutrition out of the calories consumed and find a balance between eating and physical activity.

Sounds good, doesn't it? Indeed, it does represent a modest step forward in the painfully slow process of forcing big government and big business to address the nutrition issue. But there is some bad news. These guidelines are supposed to be about diet, so why are they talking about exercise? Emphasizing weight loss conveniently puts the responsibility for dietary change on the individual, and in so doing evades reining in the food industry's multibillion-dollar budget for marketing and promoting unhealthy foods.

Until we are given clear, honest, unbiased information, the nation's health will continue to suffer. Imagine the guidelines said, "Stop eating McDonald's, Burger King and Taco Bell." Now that's something Americans would be able to understand, but instead of getting this specific, the guidelines recommend avoiding certain ingredients, such as trans fats. Food labels disguise these fats with names most people don't recognize, and therefore can't avoid. Partially hydrogenated oils, for instance, which are in almost all commercially packaged junk food such as margarine, most peanut butter and cookies, are trans fats. How are we supposed to know that? The guidelines certainly don't tell us.

In spite of strong objections from the sugar industry, the new guidelines contain advice to lessen sugar intake, especially in soft drinks and fruit juices. But the report stops short of telling people plainly to eat less sugar. And, of course, no one in Washington would dream of saying bluntly to the public, "Stop drinking so much Coke and Pepsi. They're loaded with sugar and it's bad for you!"

Dr. Walter Willett, chair of the Department of Nutrition at Harvard School of Public Health, author of the book *Eat, Drink and Be Healthy,* and guest lecturer at our institute, also criticizes the new guidelines. He created a scorecard, ranking who will benefit the most from the new guidelines. "Big dairy" came out on top with a score of 10 points. "Big beef" came second with eight points. The public's health came third with six points. "Big sugar" ended up with two points. Because their interests were protected, two of the most powerful groups in the food industry—dairy and beef—did better than the public, but sugar came in last as the national scapegoat for the obesity problem.

In 1967 the U.S. Senate Select Committee first tried to warn the public that excessive consumption of red meat and dairy causes obesity and serious illness. But the power of the lobby groups gagged the politicians and government, and they continue to do so today while both industries benefit from substantial government subsidies. In fact, the USDA's recommended intake of dairy actually increases in the new guidelines, despite recent evidence linking dairy to breast cancer, a disease that hits one out of every nine American women. There is absolutely no mention of any adverse side effects from dairy, such as asthma, allergies, digestive upset, osteoporosis, cardiovascular disease, vitamin D toxicity, iron deficiency and food allergies. "Dairy is clearly not an essential part of diet," says Willett. "Most of the world doesn't consume dairy as an adult, and if you need some extra calcium you can get it as a supplement."

Willett praises the guidelines' suggestion to increase whole grain consumption because these grains take longer to digest and break down more slowly into glucose. They also contain naturally occurring vitamins and minerals. But most shoppers don't even know what a whole grain is, or how to distinguish brown rice from Uncle Ben's white rice, or plain oatmeal from Cheerios with added sugar and salt. Try going into a supermarket and asking the employees where to find whole grains. I bet they won't be able to tell you. Ask where the soda, cookies or ice cream is, however, and they'll immediately point to aisle upon aisle dedicated to these products. Even natural food stores now have large areas for "healthy" versions of these junk foods.

The government falls short again in educating the public about how to identify whole grains. The USDA website lists whole wheat flour, bulgur, oatmeal, rye bread, whole cornmeal and brown rice as examples. Yes, brown rice is a whole grain, but the others are not; they are processed foods made from whole grains. Some suggestions by the USDA to get more whole grains are to eat whole grain cereals, whole grain muffins, whole grain bread or crackers, cookies made from whole grain flour, oatmeal or a whole grain snack chip, such as baked tortilla chips. Not one of these is a whole food.

In order to eat the recommended six to 11 servings of grain products per day, we are told by the USDA to have one cup whole wheat flakes or half an English muffin for breakfast, one turkey sandwich on two slices of whole wheat bread for lunch, nine three-ring pretzels for an afternoon snack, one cup white rice and one dinner roll with dinner, and three cups popped popcorn as a late snack. These are all processed foods, most of which have added salt and sugar, and they are stripped of the nutrients contained in an actual whole grain. The guidelines recommend many products made from wheat, but fail to mention that some Americans have allergies and intolerances to wheat and wheat products. There is a section on the website called "Less common whole grains," where they list amaranth, millet and quinoa—not exactly an endorsement for these healthful and unknown foods. They have no space for kasha, barley, kamut, whole oats or spelt.

The guidelines do not explain the benefits of eating an actual whole grain as opposed to a processed whole grain product like pasta, bread or crackers. There is no mention of where to buy, how to cook or how to prepare genuine whole grains. You would think the USDA would do a better job of teaching people about the foods they are telling them to eat. The way this information is presented speaks volumes about the extent to which the government wants as little as possible to do with shaking up the status quo.

• • • MyPyramid • • •

To accompany the new guidelines, the USDA released MyPyramid in April 2005. The original pyramid has been turned on its side and divided into six different colored sections to represent the food groups: grains, vegetables, fruits, milk, meat and beans, and oils. A stick figure climbing stairs to the left of the pyramid illustrates the importance of exercise, and matches the new slogan, "Steps to a Healthier You." The design is colorful, but the pyramid itself contains little information about what to eat. For instance, the vegetable section is about the same size as the milk section, so does that mean you should consume the same amounts of milk and vegetables? In order to find out what and how much you should actually eat, you must visit the MyPyramid website.

Upon entering the site, you are asked to input your age, gender and activity level. Based on this personal information, you are presented with "customized" recommendations—one of the 12 pyramids designed by the USDA, each eating plan meant to cater to the individual. The idea is that one size doesn't fit all, and our food intake depends on our lifestyle. In theory this is great, but at a closer look, the advice in all 12 is very similar: three whole grains each day, vary your veggies, get your calcium-rich foods, go lean on protein and limit calories from extra sugar and fat.

MyPyramid promotes the idea that we can eat a lot and whatever we like as long as we are exercising every day. Calories in, calories out: a concept that benefits both the food and the exercise industries. Even

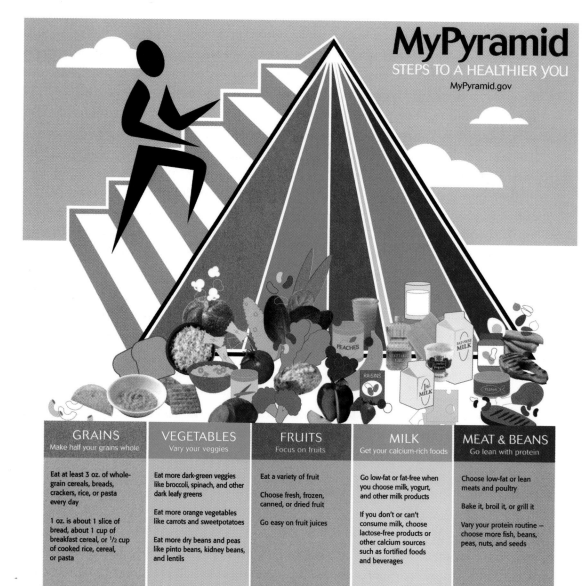

MyPyramid

STEPS TO A HEALTHIER YOU

MyPyramid.gov

GRAINS	VEGETABLES	FRUITS	MILK	MEAT & BEANS
Make half your grains whole	Vary your veggies	Focus on fruits	Get your calcium-rich foods	Go lean with protein
Eat at least 3 oz. of whole-grain cereals, breads, crackers, rice, or pasta every day

1 oz. is about 1 slice of bread, about 1 cup of breakfast cereal, or ½ cup of cooked rice, cereal, or pasta | Eat more dark-green veggies like broccoli, spinach, and other dark leafy greens

Eat more orange vegetables like carrots and sweetpotatoes

Eat more dry beans and peas like pinto beans, kidney beans, and lentils | Eat a variety of fruit

Choose fresh, frozen, canned, or dried fruit

Go easy on fruit juices | Go low-fat or fat-free when you choose milk, yogurt, and other milk products

If you don't or can't consume milk, choose lactose-free products or other calcium sources such as fortified foods and beverages | Choose low-fat or lean meats and poultry

Bake it, broil it, or grill it

Vary your protein routine — choose more fish, beans, peas, nuts, and seeds |

For a 2,000-calorie diet, you need the amounts below from each food group. To find the amounts that are right for you, go to MyPyramid.gov.

| Eat 6 oz. every day | Eat 2½ cups every day | Eat 2 cups every day | Get 3 cups every day;
for kids aged 2 to 8, it's 2 | Eat 5½ oz. every day |

Find your balance between food and physical activity

- Be sure to stay within your daily calorie needs.
- Be physically active for at least 30 minutes most days of the week.
- About 60 minutes a day of physical activity may be needed to prevent weight gain.
- For sustaining weight loss, at least 60 to 90 minutes a day of physical activity may be required.
- Children and teenagers should be physically active for 60 minutes every day, or most days.

Know the limits on fats, sugars, and salt (sodium)

- Make most of your fat sources from fish, nuts, and vegetable oils.
- Limit solid fats like butter, stick margarine, shortening, and lard, as well as foods that contain these.
- Check the Nutrition Facts label to keep saturated fats, trans fats, and sodium low.
- Choose food and beverages low in added sugars. Added sugars contribute calories with few, if any, nutrients.

MyPyramid.gov
STEPS TO A HEALTHIER YOU

U.S. Department of Agriculture
Center for Nutrition Policy and Promotion
April 2005
CNPP-15

USDA

USDA is an equal opportunity provider and employer.

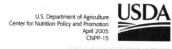

if all Americans exercised 30 minutes each day it wouldn't be enough to counteract the amount of sugar and meat we are eating. And most people do not exercise 30 minutes every single day. It's inaccurate and unhelpful to build a food pyramid based on this premise. A better plan would be to build a food pyramid for people who exercise zero minutes a day since that is what the majority of Americans are doing.

In the spirit of looking at the positives and negatives of all dietary theories, as we do at our school, I'd like to highlight the improvements made by the USDA since the previous Food Guide Pyramid as well. MyPyramid mentions the importance of eating both leafy green vegetables and whole grains, two health-providing foods that the old pyramid was missing. Also, I firmly believe that there is no one right diet for everyone, and MyPyramid acknowledges this concept by having the 12 different pyramids.

Sadly, however, the USDA still has a long way to go before making real waves in helping the public understand how to eat well. Directing people to a website for nutrition advice makes the issue more complex than it needs to be. It is not difficult to clearly state what foods are beneficial and detrimental to health. Vegetables are the food missing most from the average American diet, and the most commonly consumed vegetable products in America are French fries, potato chips and ketchup. People need to be told clearly to eat more vegetables, eat more whole foods, drink more water, eat less or no fast food, drink less or no soda and stop eating sugar all day long. And these recommendations need to be financially supported by the government.

• • • Government Policy • • •

Due to political campaign contributions and powerful political lobbies, the government will not state the truth about nutrition. Politicians say the money they receive does not influence policy, but why would companies give money if this were true? Corporations are not known for their generosity. Politicians need a lot of money to get elected, and food and drug companies have that kind of money. If you're McDonald's, General Mills, Kraft, Nestlé or Hershey, it helps to have friends in Washington, D.C. who make the food laws and guidelines.

Another important practice to understand when it comes to food and government is subsidization. Since the 1920s, American farmers have received support from the government in order to keep themselves in business, stabilize crop prices and keep the cost of food down for the American public. Wheat, soybeans and corn are the most highly subsidized crops. Products made from these crops, such as high fructose corn syrup and hydrogenated fats created from soybeans, provide a cheap way to add flavor to packaged foods. The overproduction of these crops encouraged by government subsidies leads to a surplus, and this causes the prices of packaged junk food, fast food, corn-fed beef and pork, and soft drinks sweetened with high fructose corn syrup to drop. These less nutritious foods are cheaper, and tempting to those of us who live on a budget. Farmers who receive support to grow these crops often disregard the cultivation of fruits, vegetables and other grains. In short, these subsidies contribute to the obesity epidemic by making unhealthy foods cheaper and easily available.

In looking at the new pyramid, it's odd to see that the government is not subsidizing foods they recommend we eat. Less than one-tenth of a dollar that is put into subsidizing and promoting foods through the USDA goes towards fruits and vegetables. Why aren't vegetables, fruits and whole grains heavily subsidized so they can be cheaper and more accessible, helping people to follow the government's own nutritional guidelines?

The U.S. is a wealthy country. Our annual budget is $2.5 trillion. Guess how much of that money is going towards promoting the new pyramid? Zero. There is no budget. Why would a wealthy country in the middle of an obesity epidemic not allocate resources to help its citizens with diet and nutrition?

• • • Supersized Nation • • •

One way to view the connection between diet and health in dramatic, colorful and hilarious terms is to watch Morgan Spurlock's movie *Supersize Me*, in which the filmmaker eats three meals a day at McDonald's for a month to study the impact of fast food on the body. Spurlock's intention in making the movie was to create a wake-up call for Americans.

He painfully discovered that eating these foods all day, every day, for 90 meals in a row made him very sick. By the end of this experiment, Spurlock had gained 24 pounds, his cholesterol had skyrocketed 65 points, his blood-fat levels were sent soaring and, in one of his doctor's words, his liver turned into pate. He also felt physically and emotionally addicted to the food, despite repercussions of headaches, chest pain, mood swings, exhaustion and depression. It took him many months on his girlfriend's special healing diet to get his blood levels back to normal after the experiment was over. Regaining normal weight took even longer. We are proud to say that his fiancé, Alex Jamieson, is a graduate of our school.

• • • Just Say No to Drugs • • •

The pharmaceutical industry is by far the most profitable one in the U.S. Recorded profits of the top drug companies continue to rank high above those of other industries, including commercial banking. In 2002 the top 10 drug companies made a higher profit than all the other 490 businesses on the Fortune 500 list combined. Meanwhile, the public is guided by advertising and doctors to believe they need more medication, and the prices for these drugs are rising. In her book *The Truth About Drug Companies: How They Deceive Us and What to Do About It*, Dr. Marcia Angell, a Harvard lecturer and former *New England Journal of Medicine* editor-in-chief, argues that drug companies must find a better, less expensive way of doing business.

According to Angell, 1980 was the year when profit-making really took off. Until then, research was funded by taxpayers and those funds were available to any company that wanted to use them. Legislation introduced in 1980 allowed public tax money, university medical researchers and big drug companies to form an alliance. Suddenly, pure research disappeared. Universities could patent their discoveries and grant exclusive licenses to drug companies.

Not long afterwards, Congress passed another series of laws extending monopoly rights for brand-name drugs to a total of 14 years, another big win for the pharmaceutical industry. This allows companies to sell competition for 14 years, enabling them to charge exorbitant prices. Once this time period expires, generic copies of the drug are sold and profits decline dramatically.

As profits escalated, so did the political clout of drug companies. By 1990, the industry had unprecedented control over its own fortunes. If it didn't like something about the Food and Drug Administration, the federal agency that is supposed to regulate the industry, it could change it through direct pressure or friends in Congress.

These new policies led to a transformation in the ethos of medical school. Professors and faculty members began to wonder, If they were the medical experts, why weren't they seeing financial benefits? Feeling the lack, medical schools put more resources into searching for commercial opportunities and welcomed big sponsorships from the pharmaceutical industry. This strongly impacted the education in medical school. Future doctors may enter medical school with idealistic notions about helping society, preventing illness and making America a healthier place, but many of them leave believing that modern drugs are the easiest and quickest way to cure any symptom.

America does not have to deal with health and medicine this way. As I mentioned before, in the ancient Chinese medical system patients paid the doctor when they were healthy and stopped paying him when they fell sick. If the doctor wanted payments to resume, he had to get his patients well again. The whole emphasis was on creating and maintaining a general state of wellness. It was the doctor's job to make sure people stayed healthy, rather than coming into the picture only when they became ill, as happens now.

If the income of medical professionals today depended on keeping people healthy, the word would go out like lightning, resonating loudly and clearly from every doctor's office. Doctors would be urging their patients to stay away from junk foods and directing them to the fruits and vegetables section of their local natural food store instead. Surgeons would protest in the soda aisle and nurses would petition against television commercials and highway billboards seducing small children to visit Playland.

If we want to be healthy, we need to eat nutritious foods. It really isn't such a difficult thing to do, but, unfortunately, there aren't many people around who are willing to help us do it. The food industry, drug companies, politicians, civil servants and even the medical profession all have strong vested interests in keeping you unhealthy. In one way or another, almost all the sources of information and advice we would expect to support our quest for overall health are contaminated for reasons of financial gain. Face it, America. Being healthy just isn't good for business!

• • • The American Dietetic Association • • •

With nearly 70,000 members, the American Dietetic Association (ADA) claims to be the nation's largest organization of food and nutrition professionals. Founded in Cleveland, Ohio, in 1917 by a group of women dedicated to helping the government conserve food and improve the public's health and nutrition during World War I, the organization's mission is "leading the future of dietetics," with ADA members serving the public as "the most valued source" of good advice about food and nutrition, with a whole-hearted commitment "to helping people enjoy healthy lives." Could anything sound more wholesome?

When the Ohio state legislature passed a law creating the Ohio Board of Dietetics in 1987, it made sense to effectively prevent anyone from giving advice on nutrition except members of the ADA. After all, we don't want unqualified people giving advice. This would have worked if the new board had protected the public from poor nutrition advice instead of protecting its own dietitians from competition. And even this would have been okay for most Americans, remaining a problem only for Ohio citizens, but the ADA spread its tentacles all over the country, trying to get state-by-state legislation to exclude everyone other than their affiliates from giving nutritional advice.

Problems in Ohio began shortly after the law was passed. The board received national attention as a result of its interference with the activities of a well-known nutritionist from California who had intended to present an ongoing education program at an Ohio hospital. This was followed by increasingly stringent rules and regulations—even public speeches about nutrition were prohibited—combined with aggressive action by the board against its competitors.

Over a six-year period, beginning in 1996, the board went after 795 people, but made a serious tactical error when it turned its guns on Dr. Pamela Popper, a nutrition counselor with two PhDs, author of several books and founder of The Wellness Forum, a chain of health and wellness centers located throughout the U.S. Popper not only fought the board and the ADA, but also vigorously campaigned to expose their practices and roll back many aspects of the law. Popper made people aware that dietetics is only a small part of nutrition theory, and publicized the fact that the ADA is heavily funded by the food industry, receiving millions of dollars a year from agricultural organizations and corporations that manufacture food and food additives.

According to Popper, the ADA's positions on a number of health- and nutrition-related subjects are, literally, bought and paid for. "You can't take $50,000 a year from the sugar association and say bad things about sugar," she explained. "This organization controls the educational programming and registration of the thousands of dietitians in the U.S," she added. "It is my personal opinion that the influence of industry on the practice of dietitians is one of the reasons why nutrition in institutions such as hospitals, schools and nursing homes continues to be abominable."

While sympathizing with Popper and admiring her courage to take on the ADA, I would not have felt so strongly about the activities of this group had I not personally felt their influence at a meeting in Albany, New York, where I suddenly found myself being questioned in a critical manner about the credentials of our institute. At the meeting was an official of the state health department who told me, "We are looking at legislation to ensure that only professionals can advise people about diet." By chance, the main spokesman of the team happened to be suffering from a heavy cold and kept reaching for a box of tissues, so halfway through the discussion, just to underline the absurdity of the situation, I jokingly said to her, "You know, I could tell you what to do for your cold, but I might get arrested."

Really, the story of the ADA is just part of the long history of commerce in this country, in which each interest group tries to destroy the opposition in order to create a monopoly for itself, thereby acquiring more power, status and profit. This raises an important question. If we cannot trust any of these groups, including the dietitians, to give us good advice about health, nutrition and diet, whom can we trust?

• • • The Turning Point • • •

You are the only person who can make yourself healthy. The first step is to slow down, listen to your body and understand yourself from the inside out. Once you understand this and get yourself well, you will likely be inspired to reach out to your family and friends to relieve their needless suffering. Now is the time to make a difference. If we all stand up and speak up for what we know to be true, we will dramatically improve the current healthcare system in this country. And when America changes, the world will change.

exercises

1. Supermarket Field Trip

Go to your local supermarket with a friend or family member, walk around and look into people's shopping carts, noticing what they are buying. Supermarkets are where 90% of Americans get their food. This should give you a good understanding of what people are eating.

Write down the most common food items you see in people's carts:

_____

_____

_____

_____

Imagine, how would you feel if you were eating these foods?

_____

_____

_____

_____

2. Examine MyPyramid

Go to www.mypyramid.gov. What makes sense to you?

The set up is easy for everyone to follow. They recomend a diet based on a person's size & activity level. There is a deffinate undertone of "eat more vegies"

What doesn't?

Milk has its own category? (why?) There is no question about if women are pregnant or nursing. The "whole grains" they talk about are not whole grains.

Can you locate misinformation or disinformation?

Lack of dairy alternatives. No explanation of what whole foods really are. It implies that a healthy diet must contain animal products.

Imagine that you have been appointed the supreme head of the USDA. What changes would you make?

_____

_____

3. Watch *Supersize Me*

As you watch Spurlock's progress, reflect on the times that you ate fast food and how it made you feel. Begin to notice how different foods affect your mood, energy levels and body.

4. Trustworthy Professionals

Make a list of the "experts" in health and nutrition that you trust the most:

The ones who are healthy/happy themselves.
Michelle Linet, Suzanne Tully, Mo, Dr. Fountain

Is there any expert you would trust with your life?

I don't know

Where has your most faithful, useful and solid health and nutrition information come from?

My intuition combined with suggestions from various aquaintances and books like "Nutritional healing", also from the people @ Rainbow Natural Remedies

What would help you become a trustworthy expert?

Learning to listen to my body's needs and being disciplined enough to act on them. And then helping others find the confidence in themselves to do the same.

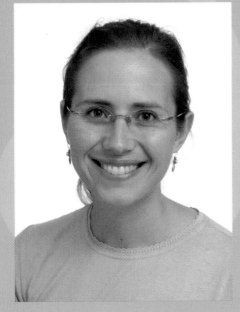

my first year in medical school, I noticed a disconnect between who I was and what I was learning. I struggled with managing the stress, workload and competition of the medical school system. I wondered how I was going to get through the next few years. When I found the Integrative Nutrition magazine, I immediately read it cover to cover. Here was the missing piece to my education!

Being a student at Integrative Nutrition was an experience that changed my personal and professional life. They addressed spirituality, movement, career and relationship. I was amazed and overjoyed with the unique whole-body teaching approach. I never knew learning could be so much fun! I came to appreciate the healing relationship by being both counselor and counselee. I came away with a practical knowledge of how to eat and live healthy, and how to share that with others. Most of us know what to do to feel better. Learning how to do it has been one of my greatest gifts.

The school teaches many different dietary theories in an unbiased manner with a strong emphasis on there being no right diet. Thus, I learned how to listen to my own body and not whatever rigid "rules" my mind thinks are best. As a result, I am much healthier and happier. My organizational and teaching skills have improved dramatically as a result of this course. I am confident in my abilities to provide quality services to patients from both a compassionate and business perspective, which complements the strong clinical training I am receiving at medical school.

Rather than waiting until I finish my residency to start helping people, I am now giving lectures and workshops to medical students on how to balance work, stress and eating. My fellow students are really responsive to it and want to know more. There is a desperateness for this information; and, unfortunately, it's not covered in our medical training.

In medical school, I am learning how to treat illness. I am passionate about becoming the best possible doctor I can be. Yet I fundamentally believe there are many things people can do to prevent ending up in the doctor's office.

Devon Rossetto
Graduate 2004
Boston, MA
devonr@bu.edu

At Integrative Nutrition, I learned about these things, and about how to listen and help people heal themselves. As I prepare to graduate medical school this year—I am going into pediatrics—I realize how much of my success and enjoyment of life is because of my experience at Integrative Nutrition. Being able to manage time and stress, stay healthy, and stay connected with friends and family is no easy task. I am grateful for having been shown how to create my life based on what is important to me.

chapter 2

The human body is the universe in miniature.
That which cannot be found in the body,
is not to be found in the universe.
Hence the philosopher's formula,
that the universe within, reflects the universe without.
It follows therefore, that
if our knowledge of our own body could be perfect,
we would know the universe.

Mahatma Gandhi

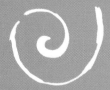

foundations of integrative nutrition

ONE OF THE MOST FUNDAMENTAL CONCEPTS that can help us embrace the beauty of an integrative approach to nutrition is bio-individuality. Nature created us as unique human beings who, while sharing many similarities, are more remarkable for the ways we differ than for the ways we are alike. While watching fad diets sweep through the country, from high carbohydrate diets in the 70s to low fat diets in the 80s to high protein diets at the dawn of the 21st century, I wondered how each of these nutrition experts could claim that their diet would work for everyone. There is no one perfect way of eating that works for everybody. We are too individualistic to all be eating the same exact food. We need to eat very differently if we have an office job or if we are a dancer; if we are a teacher or a musician; if it's Saturday night or Monday morning; if we are 25 or 55; if we're from Europe, Asia, Africa or Venus.

Numerous factors shape our bio-individuality. An example of one is our ancestry. If our ancestors were Japanese, it's most likely that we will thrive on a Japanese-type diet, high in rice, sea vegetables and fish, and that we will have difficulty digesting dairy. If our ancestors were vegetarians from India, our system will probably process grains, lentils, beans and spices more naturally than animal meat. If our ancestors were meat eaters from Holland, a diet that includes high quality meat and dairy will most likely work for us, while we may have difficulty digesting beans and grains.

Our personal tastes and preferences, natural shapes and sizes, blood types, metabolic rates and genetic backgrounds contribute to what foods will and won't work for us. So, when the experts say tomatoes are healthy or red meat is unhealthy, it is too much of a generalization. One person's food is another person's poison, and that is why fad diets do not work in the long run. They are not based on the premise that we all have different dietary needs.

Sometimes it takes millions of dollars in funding and years of research for scientists to prove what we already know. I am certain that science will soon discover diet needs to be based on bio-individuality. We already see it happening, to some extent, with the USDA's new Dietary Guidelines and the 12 different pyramids. This is just the beginning.

• • • The Laboratory of Your Body • • •

Fortunately, you already have free, 24-hour access to the world's most sophisticated laboratory for testing how food affects your body and your health. Where is that lab? You're living in it. Your body is a sophisticated bio-computer. By learning to listen to your body and developing an understanding of what foods it needs and when it needs them, you will discover what is best for you.

If you doubt your ability to do this, remember that your body is super smart. Your heart never misses a beat and your lungs are always breathing in and out. Even if you break up with your boyfriend, girl-friend, wife or husband, even if you receive traumatic news, your heart's four little chambers go right on pumping and your lungs continue to expand and contract. You can trust your body. It has evolved helpful instincts over thousands of years.

Just as a tree will always lean towards light, humans and animals know instinctively how and where to get food that is best for them. You may have noticed that animals don't read nutrition books. Their bodies contain a built-in program that tells them which plants to eat and which to avoid, or, if they're predators, which animals to kill when they're hungry. They heal themselves when they are sick, usually by resting a lot and eating very little until the sickness passes.

Our heritage has given us the same instincts. Until a short time ago, these instincts guided the entire human population. We knew what to eat; we grew and gathered locally available food; we learned from our elders how to prepare it and we cooked and ate together as a tribe or family. In more recent decades, we've become distracted. All kinds of foods that are not fit for human consumption have been invented, packaged and presented in brightly colored containers to entice us.

In order to override our natural instincts and have us eat these convenience foods, corporations have spent tons of money on marketing. Here I'd like to introduce Joshua's Law of Advertising. It goes like this: The less likely humans are to eat a certain food, the more heavily it will be advertised. The most heav-ily advertised products are cigarettes, alcohol, junk food and fast foods because, given half a chance to think about it, the average person would never touch the stuff. The message has to be repeatedly blasted into us until we find ourselves saying, "I have to have that!" Nobody wakes up in the morning and thinks, "Today I think I'll really mess up my body and eat garbage." But this is happening because we are so influenced by advertising that we have lost touch with our bodies' instincts.

[handwritten margin note: Joshua's Law of Advertising]

If you give yourself time to explore the laboratory of your body, you will be surprised how responsive, sophisticated and intelligent it is. It is a highly sensitive organism that wants to be healthy and wants to communicate with you about the food you supply it.

• • • The Lost Art of Listening • • •

Listening is at a premium. Many of us listen to the voices in our heads, our minds, to society, and at times we listen to our hearts, but very few of us actually listen to our bodies. Our bodies are constantly sending us messages that we overlook. If we have dark circles under our eyes, it may be a sign of exhaustion and our body telling us to slow down and get some rest. If we are having digestive issues, such as constipation and bloating, our body may be telling us that something we are eating, or the way we are eating it, is not appropriate. Most people ignore these messages until they are unbearable, and that's when they go to the doctor for medications and operations.

Just as we rarely listen to our bodies, it's also infrequent that we listen to people. Most people live in their heads, thinking about what they have to do tomorrow, what happened yesterday or an hour ago, pretty much anything except being in the present moment. It's very rare to have a conversation with someone who actually listens to what you're saying, without interruption and without judgment. Have you ever been to a party where someone asked you a question and then didn't even listen to a word of your answer? This happens all the time. It is equally unusual that we listen to another person without interrupting them, judging or thinking about what we're going to say next. I encourage you when talking with others to really listen to what they are saying. Put all thoughts about yourself out of your head and be there for them. It will greatly improve the quality of your communication.

We are all starving to be really listened to. Healing occurs when this happens. It occurs when we hear the profound messages that come through those around us, from our bodies and from food.

• • • Food-Mood Journal • • •

One of the best ways to listen to your body and to learn how it reacts to food is to create a Food-Mood Journal. Start by writing what you eat and how you feel afterwards. Be sure to write how you feel immediately after and how you feel a few hours later. As you know, you may feel good right after eating candy or drinking coffee, but two hours later it is often a different story. For example, you may write, "I had tea first thing this morning, and I felt good. I had coffee at eleven and still felt okay, but the second cup of coffee after lunch put me over the top." Or you may notice, "I had too much animal meat today and felt lethargic." Or, perhaps, "Every time I eat bread, my stomach hurts." Or, "Yesterday I had a nice spinach and lentil soup, but wanted something more. I had a small piece of chocolate for dessert and felt satisfied." Soon you know what energizes and what drains you. Certain foods will give you gas; certain foods will stop you from sleeping well; other foods will enhance your ability to concentrate at work. The average person doesn't see the connection between their food and their mood, but once you make the connection, there is no going back.

It's surprising how deeply food affects us. In relationships, we often get irritated and blame our partner when actually it's our own mood swings that are causing the disturbance. We are going up and down like a yo-yo and as soon as we come into a nutritional state of balance, suddenly our love partner turns out to be a wonderful person. Again, I simply encourage you to notice, explore, experiment and determine what works for you.

• • • Energy of Food • • •

When increasing awareness around the food you are eating, it is important to understand that all foods have their own unique energy. Steve Gagné, a health educator for 25 years, guest lecturer at our institute and author of *Energetics of Food: Encounters with Your Most Intimate Relationship*, did an original study on the subject. His book goes into great detail over the distinct qualities of many different foods. Where they grow, how they grow and when they grow all add to these qualities. When we eat food, we not only assimilate its nutrients and vitamins, but also its energy. By using this concept, we can choose foods that create the energy we are seeking in our lives.

There is a theory in nutrition that a protein is a protein is a protein. The current food pyramid says meat, poultry, fish, beans, eggs and nuts are basically the same. In America, the main source of protein is cow. People eat beef from cows and dairy from cows. It's a large part of most people's daily diet. Beef and dairy are available in pretty much every restaurant and increasingly, Americans look like cows, with big, beefy bodies and wide eyes. We look much different than people whose cultures eat mostly rice, fish or fruit.

Passing character traits from animals to humans, a theory I call "cross-species transference," also results in animal-like habits. Chickens spend a lot of time and energy creating a pecking order to establish who is higher on the social scale. They are generally noisy, nervous, frenetic creatures and are cooped up in small, overcrowded cages when raised in factory farms. This may be the perfect food for someone who is very quiet, lethargic and wants to be more social, but for a high-strung, stressed-out person, chicken is probably not a good food choice.

My enthusiasm for these insights, which may seem esoteric and difficult to prove scientifically, stems from the fact that I developed a knack for spotting the influence of specific animal foods on people, and was so impressed by the results that I embarked on a long-term study. When someone in my class had a pronounced, beak-like nose and a tense, nervous disposition, I'd ask, "Have you eaten a lot of chicken?" Sure enough, nine times out of 10, the answer would be yes. Or, at a social event, I'd bump into someone strong and muscular, with a red face. Again, when I asked, "Do you eat a lot of beef?", the answer would be yes.

One client had me stumped. Even though I was deeply engrossed in visual diagnosis and cross-species transference at the time, and doing well in guessing the animal diets of other people, I could not figure him out. He was a huge guy, with very large ears, a big, round nose, thick arms and legs, and small eyes. Yet he was not loud or aggressive. He was very gentle and shy. To be honest, he looked a bit like an elephant, but I dismissed this idea as impossible. As the consultation continued, I asked, "What was the animal food you ate growing up?"

He looked at me and said, "Elephant."

I practically fell off my chair. I raised my eyebrows and said, "Really? You're kidding!"

He said, "No, I grew up in South Africa on a forest reserve."

He explained that the local elephant population had to be culled from time to time to avoid environmental devastation, and because this meat was plentiful, free and wholesome, his family developed the habit of eating elephant meat. At this point in time, I became convinced of the strong correlation between animal foods and human development.

The energy of plant foods also has a powerful effect on us. Greens like kale, collards and bok choy are tender, with delicate leaves reaching up towards the sun, soaking up the chlorophyll. They are great for lifting the spirit. Root vegetables, like carrots and burdock, have a strong downward energy, great for when we need grounding.

Once you open your eyes to this information, it's amazing to discover the extent that it's true. We are entrained by the food we eat. Our bodies absorb the qualities passed on to us by the contents of our food choices, especially when the food in question is meat. What impresses me is how incredibly sensitive and adaptable the human body can be. We can change our moods, our bodies and our minds by making small changes in our daily diet. Understanding the flexible nature of your own biological organism will be encouragement for you to explore and experiment with different foods. Your body will respond to the changes you make, and you will feel the difference. Just give it a try.

• • • Food Quality • • •

One of the most profound ways to experience the energetic nature of food is to begin to notice the properties of organic food. Have you noticed that organic food can feel more vital? Cleaner? More potent? Originally, all foods were "organic"—grown and prepared without pesticides, herbicides, chemical fertilizers, hormones, irradiation to prevent spoilage or microwave cooking. Foods were unrefined and whole. Since World War II and the dawn of chemical farming and food processing, the soils and foods of much of the world have been depleted of minerals and other nutrients.

Our food these days, whether of vegetable or animal origin, is not only deficient in nutrients, but also full of pollutants and farm chemicals. The modern denaturing of foods through massive refining and chemical treatment deeply affects their life force, making it difficult to foster equilibrium and health.

Pesticides, which have been shown to cause cancer as well as liver, kidney and blood diseases, must be dealt with by the immune system. As pesticides get lodged and build in our tissues, the immune system becomes weakened, allowing other carcinogens and pathogens to affect our health.

Fresh, organic produce contains more vitamins, minerals, enzymes and other micronutrients than intensively farmed produce. Organic produce is not covered in chemicals. The average conventionally grown apple has 20 to 30 artificial chemicals on its skin, even after rinsing. Organic produce also tastes better. Fruit and vegetables have more flavor. Experiment with an organic carrot and a conventionally grown carrot. The organic one will undoubtedly taste sweeter.

Even though organic is usually more expensive, the few extra cents you pay for organic food may save you hundreds if not thousands of dollars in future doctors bills.

• • • Metabolic Rate • • •

Metabolism is the rate at which we convert food into energy, in the form of calories, and burn it as fuel in our cells. Knowing your personal metabolic rate is useful when gauging the quantity of food your digestive system can process. Energy cannot be destroyed, and food is energy, so the energy of your food is either used or stored. Depending on your metabolic rate, your body may quickly convert calories to energy, or it may do it slowly, storing the extra calories. You may recall that as a teenager you could wolf down a burger, fries, milkshake and ice cream all in one meal, without any indigestion or tightening of your jeans. That's because young people are still growing, have fast metabolic rates and burn calories more quickly than adults.

Some people are born with a fast metabolism that stays with them through adulthood, and can burn up the calories no matter what they eat or how old they are, keeping them rail thin their whole lives. Most of us, however, follow the norm of a gradually slowing metabolic rate, with increasing tendency towards storing extra fat. It's helpful to recognize and accept the change as it is happening. Then you can tailor your food intake accordingly and keep your body in shape.

The good news is that you can influence your metabolic rate. There are simple, easy ways to speed it up, and perhaps more importantly, keep it from slowing down. Whether walking, bicycling, jogging, swimming, playing tennis or dancing, any activity that boosts your heart rate for 20 to 30 minutes or more increases your metabolic rate, keeping those calories burning for a long time after you've stopped. The more your muscles are utilized, the more energy you burn, so staying in shape through weight training is also a good way to maintain a vigorous metabolism and keep off the extra pounds.

There are two nervous systems involved in metabolism: the sympathetic nervous system, known as "fight or flight," and the parasympathetic, known as "rest and digest." The sympathetic system inhibits digestion. As our caveman ancestors discovered, you don't want to waste energy processing food while you're running away from a saber-toothed tiger. The parasympathetic nervous system directs blood to the digestive tract and makes sure food is actively digested. It also maintains blood pressure, heart rate and breathing rate at a low level.

As far as metabolic rates are concerned, people may be divided into three general types:
Fast Burner or Protein types tend to be frequently hungry, crave fatty, salty foods and don't do well on low calorie diets. These people benefit from a higher protein intake.

Slow Burner or Carbo types generally have relatively weak appetites, a high tolerance for sweets and problems with weight control. They require a higher percentage of carbohydrates.

Mixed types generally have average appetites and moderate cravings for sweets and starchy foods. For them, the ideal diet is a balanced combination of protein and carbohydrates.

Discovering your metabolic type can be done by answering questionnaires or taking simple medical tests. There are many websites where you can take a free metabolic test, one of which I will mention at the end of this chapter. If it seems too confusing and complicated, don't worry. All you really need to observe is how your own body responds to the food you give it. People are different, and getting to know your own body is an essential first step in discovering your personal way to keep healthy.

Metabolism is a good way to demonstrate that no one diet is right for all of us. You may know people who can eat processed carbohydrates, such as bread and pasta, and stay very thin while you gain weight on such a diet. It's not because carbohydrates are evil or your body isn't as good as those of your friends, it just shows that you metabolize these foods differently. You'd probably do better on a high protein diet with lots of fresh vegetables and some whole grains. Knowing what foods you metabolize best will help you to choose foods that make you feel good and support your health.

Our knowledge about the human organism is constantly increasing. Yesterday's nutritional truths become today's discarded, disproved hypotheses. For decades it was believed that to lose weight all we needed to do was cut calories. Simple, right? But there's an unfortunate side effect. When you cut out fattening foods and discipline yourself to follow a meager list of acceptable foods, your body doesn't know you've begun a diet program. It's never heard of Atkins, South Beach or the Zone. Instead, it digs into its cellular memory and concludes, "There's a famine and this body is in imminent danger of starving to death!" So, instead of burning fat, your metabolism goes into energy reserve by storing calories, trying to preserve fat cells and lowering your metabolic rate, making weight loss more difficult. Your body strengthens its absorption abilities and learns to squeeze every last nutrient out of the available food you are giving it. As a result, when you return to a normal diet you are likely to gain weight more quickly than before. The solution to this problem involves making permanent, healthy, long-term changes to your diet and lifestyle.

• • • Hunger and Binging • • •

You may like to consider the idea, almost heretical in this day and age, that it's okay to be hungry now and then. I'm not talking about a drastic form of starvation dieting, but just an experiment to see how it feels. It's not going to kill you, and it may make life more interesting. Most people avoid hunger like the plague and many have developed habits of overeating and eating when not hungry just to avoid ever being hungry. When we habitually overeat, a high proportion of our available energy is always directed towards digestion. If we eat when we are not hungry, we are not going to digest that food very well.

On the other hand, many people today try to diet and go hungry all day. This creates a backlash, which I call the binge eaters diet. These well-intentioned people decide to eat as little as possible in an attempt to lose weight. They skip breakfast, go off to work, maybe grab a mid-morning cup of coffee to keep going, and then settle for a salad for lunch. Somehow they make it through the afternoon, but by the time they get home in the evening they discover, naturally, that they are ravenous. Maybe the hectic activity of the workday distracted them from urgent messages emanating from their stomachs, but as they slow down it just clicks, "Oh my god, I am so hungry!" Then they overeat and start the cycle over again the next morning because the food from last night's binge is still filling their stomachs and they are not hungry for breakfast. *[margin note: Negative effects of hunger dieting]*

I am not a believer in trying to override natural instincts. Of course it helps to have discipline around food, but trying to control the body by using the mind is very challenging in the long term. For one thing, the head often makes mistakes. Remember when you went shopping for a new outfit, spent a lot of money but never wore the clothes you purchased? Remember when you met a good-looking guy and thought, "Wow! This is the right person for me!" and he turned out to be a jerk? Our heads make quite a lot of mistakes that our bodies don't, and one mistake your head can easily make is to think, "This is the right diet for me. I can handle this one." Our bodies don't really care what our heads think. Our bodies are built to survive and thrive. Your head can say, "I am not eating this food," and your body may cooperate for a while, but at some point it will start murmuring quiet messages like, "Hmm, well, we definitely need more fat in the diet." The next thing you know, you're holding an empty pint of ice cream in your hand.

Learning to listen to your body is essential because the longer you ignore it, the more extreme the backlash will be. Like a crying child who needs attention and uses increasingly extreme measures to get it, the body will do what it has to in order to get you to notice it. If you don't listen, your cravings will get stronger or disease will occur. The sooner you listen to the body, the more it will cooperate with your desires and goals. On a spiritual level, your body is the home of your consciousness, so it's good practice to respect this home, maintaining it in a clean and healthy condition.

Most nutritionists give people a list of foods to avoid and foods to eat. This is why so many people are turned off by nutrition. They think they'll have to give up their favorite foods and start eating things they don't enjoy. Taking away favorite foods from people is like taking heroin away from a heroin addict. The food is feeding them something they need. I have found that one of the most effective methods to overcome habitual consumption of readily available but unhealthy foods involves crowding these foods out.

A great place to begin such crowding out is to increase your intake of water. Buy a one-liter bottle of pure spring water, take it to work with you and sip it steadily throughout your morning. There's going to be less room inside you for coffee, black tea and soft drinks. Really, it's that simple. You will immediately begin to cut down on other liquids if you keep yourself well supplied with water. You may need a second bottle for the afternoon. People's need for water varies, so you should listen to your body in order to calculate how much you need to drink in a day. Not only will water crowd out more unhealthy drinks, it may well improve your health in other ways.

You may have heard of Dr. Fereydoon Batmanghelidj, an Iranian-born physician who gained international attention with his claim that regularly drinking water on a daily basis can treat a vast array of illnesses. "You are not sick, you are thirsty," he asserted in his best-selling 1992 book, *Your Body's Many Cries for Water*, which states that most pain and sickness is a result of chronic dehydration. Dr. Batmanghelidj concluded through years of reading and research that ordinary water prevents and cures depression, asthma, arthritis, back pain, migraines, high blood pressure, multiple sclerosis and many other illnesses. He also opposed the use of costly drugs for treating illnesses, saying that you "don't treat thirst with medication."

This insightful work grew out of years as a political prisoner in Iran. He was jailed following the Islamic Revolution in 1979. As a doctor, he was approached by other prisoners with medical problems, but was without access to medicine or drugs, so he told an ulcer patient with severe abdominal pains to drink two glasses of water. To his surprise, the patient's pain receded within minutes. This was the beginning. He later treated over 3,000 fellow prisoners who suffered from peptic ulcer, viewing the prison environment as an "ideal stress laboratory." After his release from prison in 1982, he came to the U.S. and continued his exploration of the role of water metabolism in the human body.

A majority of the American population is dehydrated. This is a significant contributor to poor health. Regularly flushing out the kidneys and bladder with water ensures that dead cells and other waste products can be expelled before they reach toxic levels. But even without these added health benefits, drinking high quality water throughout the day will effectively "crowd out" old habits of reaching for unhealthy drinks.

I'd like to touch on the controversial subject of coffee. It is simply a drug in a mug. It's an adrenaline delivery system that is presented in a slightly more attractive and socially acceptable way than having a hypodermic needle stuck in your arm. The question is, Why would a normal, healthy person in the prime of their life not be able to get through the day without an injection of adrenaline? People like to talk about the aroma and the flavor of various coffee brands just as people enthuse about certain vintage wines, and it's true to a certain point. But if you're knocking back a bottle of cabernet a day, it's not just the taste that's attracting you. It's the same with coffee. If you're drinking two or three cups a day, you have a problem. Drinking water helps to crowd out coffee, but so does healthy snacking during coffee breaks as this will boost your energy through nutrition rather than adrenaline.

As drinking water crowds out unhealthy beverages, healthy foods crowd out junk foods. Vegetables contain a great deal of nutrition, and you can eat a lot of them without risk of weight gain. The trick is to organize your daily schedule and work environment in such a way that you have access to them at all times, especially when you feel like snacking. Then you can make it to your evening meal without eating junk and inflicting damage on yourself. It takes a little practice to get to this point, but it's easily possible and I will discuss it in more detail later in chapter 9.

• • • When We Eat • • •

One Christmas while visiting India I was reminded of the significance of seasonal eating when I found myself with an oversupply of fruit. India, a subtropical country, has fruit in abundance, and I offered some to the guard outside the apartment where I was staying. Though he was a poor man, and fruit was a relative luxury for him, he thanked me and shook his head, saying, "I don't eat fruit in the wintertime because the weather gets cold at night." He'd never read a diet book, but instinctively knew that fruit is a cooling food, and he would not eat food that reduced his body temperature during a cold time of year.

Our ancestors ate seasonally because they had no choice. Fresh greens grew in spring, fruit ripened in summer, root vegetables kept them going in the fall, and people relied on animal food to get them through the winter. But then California and Florida were discovered, as well as fast road transportation and refrigerated trucks, and pretty soon we could eat more or less everything, any time we wanted. Maybe this isn't so good for us. When we have ice cream in the middle of January and barbecue on the fourth of July, it's likely to confuse the body. Eating locally grown food in accordance with the seasons will help you live in harmony with yourself, your body and the earth.

In the wintertime it's natural for a vegetarian to crave animal food because that's when the body needs to feel more solid and insulated from the cold. If you want to remain on a vegetarian diet through these cold months, it may be an interesting experiment to grill your vegetables, giving them more heat and density, and to avoid raw vegetables and salads. Thick soups—like pumpkin, peas or potato—will also help give your body a sturdy feeling.

Pay attention to the times of the day that you eat. Most of us eat habitually at regular, clocked times: before work, during the lunch break and in the evening. We may take a couple of coffee or snack breaks during the day or make a late-night visit to the fridge. Few of us pause to check whether we are really hungry, partly because eating can be entertaining and pleasant, whether socializing, alone, passing time or feeling bored.

When we eat determines how well our bodies assimilate the food. Some people follow the old proverb, "Eat breakfast like a king, lunch like a prince and dinner like a pauper." Whoever coined this saying did not foresee that many more women would be interested in nutrition than men, so we must amend this mildly chauvinistic saying to read as follows, "Eat breakfast like a queen, lunch like a princess and dinner like a pauper." (Paupers, it seems, are genderless).

Many health practitioners, dietitians and nutritionists assert that we should not eat after 7:00 pm or 8:00 pm. I agree that it's a good idea to avoid eating three hours before bed because when we sleep digestion slows, and food tends to stay in our stomachs the whole night. Some experts say we gain more weight from food we eat at night. I don't know if this is scientifically true, but I do know that I don't sleep well on a full stomach and neither do most people I know. That's a strong indication that something isn't right about it. But, again, it's something for you to explore, using your own body as your laboratory.

• • • How We Eat • • •

I have covered what we eat and when we eat, and now I'd like to address how we eat because this affects everything. People dine in odd ways, such as standing up, driving a car, in the subway, discussing business deals, watching TV, reading a book and playing video games. Eating is no longer viewed as an activity in itself, worthy of exclusive quality time. This is a pity because while we eat food we are also assimilating energetically whatever else is going on around us. The body is open and in a receiving mode, and the nourishment we take in goes beyond the vitamins and nutrients in our carrots and onions. Like it or not, we take in the general vibe of the environment in which we are eating. If we are eating in an ugly, noisy, neon-lit room, the energy of that space is going to penetrate us. We also absorb something from our surroundings if we are eating quietly in a beautiful park or by the ocean. If we are eating with people, we absorb their moods, their laughter, their complaints and their busy minds.

Families used to eat together, especially in the evenings when dad came home from work and mom finished cooking. This traditional daily ritual had a binding and beneficial effect on the family as an organic unit. As the saying goes, "A family that eats together, stays together." Sharing meals made the family more cohesive and this, in turn, kept the family interwoven with a much bigger collective fabric, a whole mind-set about the kind of society we all wanted. This mind-set is rapidly changing. Now kids eat pre-packaged microwave dinners because mom and dad are working and there's no time to prepare home-cooked meals. The food we eat affects our energy, our thoughts and our actions. If dad eats a burger for dinner, mom has a large salad and the kids eat pizza on the run, it's natural that the family will have difficulty relating to one another.

The body likes to be relaxed, inactive and in a peaceful environment when assimilating and digesting because the nature of the parasympathetic nervous system is to "rest and digest." The body doesn't want to be in "fight or flight" mode, alert for danger and unexpected events. Then it becomes tense, the eyes tighten, the heart beats faster and the blood goes to the center of the body. Proper assimilation of the nutrients in food is essential to health, and if we want this assimilation to take place, we need to calm down more when we eat.

• • • The Importance of Chewing • • •

One of the best teachers I've encountered is Lino Stanchich, a great friend, a guest lecturer at our institute and the author of *Power Eating Program: You Are How You Eat*. In his book and lectures, Lino shares the story of how his father survived a German concentration camp in World War II. The weather was extremely cold, clothing was minimal, food was sparse and all prisoners were forced to work. Many people died of starvation every day. Lino's father discovered that thoroughly chewing all his food, including snow for water, gave him increased energy. He practiced until he was chewing each bite of food 150 times and each sip of water 15 times. He shared his discovery with his fellow prisoners, but only two of them joined him in his chewing sessions. When the camp was liberated in 1945, of the original 33 prisoners only three were still alive—Lino's father and his two friends. Just four years later, Lino himself was sentenced to two years of hard labor for trying to escape from communist Yugoslavia. Amazingly, he used the lessons learned from his father to survive harsh prison conditions with energy and vitality.

Since his release Lino has spent his life deepening his understanding of nutrition and chewing. He has shared his insights with thousands of people around the world. Lino recommends sitting down to meals with joy and appreciation, saying a prayer and giving thanks. He encourages eating slowly, with awareness, and taking time to chew, breathe and perhaps listen to soothing music. Of course, he cautions against eating when working, watching television or feeling high-strung.

Many of us inhale our food. We use our fork as a shovel, putting the next bite in before we've even finished the previous one. It's part of our fast food, fast-paced culture. To help people slow down, I suggest they use chopsticks as utensils. There's only so much food these can pick up at a time. Also, putting down the fork or chopsticks between bites helps slow eating down, thereby aiding in digestion.

Chewing makes food more enjoyable as well. The sweet flavor of plant foods is released only after they have been chewed thoroughly. Complex carbohydrates start breaking down in the mouth by an enzyme in saliva known as amylase. Only by chewing the carbs thoroughly and mixing them with amylase can all of their sweetness be tasted. Sweetness, in this context, is a reward for chewing. Do you see the brilliance of the natural food system involved in this process? By utilizing our inherent craving for sweetness, nature and our body bind together to ensure we get the nutrients we need.

● ● ● Explore Your Body ● ● ●

In this chapter, I've covered a number of important foundational pieces for bringing an integrative approach to nutrition into your world. But remember, they are hypotheses to experiment with. Go out, try different foods and ways of eating. Eat at different times of the day and with different types of people. Listen to how your body responds and begin to understand the uniqueness and beauty of it. Why not enjoy it? After all, it's going to be with you for the rest of your life.

exercises

1. The Breakfast Experiment

As a way of tuning into your body and learning how to listen to its messages, explore eating a different breakfast every day for a week. Jot down what you eat and how you feel, both right after and then again two hours later.

Day 1: scrambled eggs

Day 2: scrambled tofu

Day 3: oatmeal

Day 4: boxed breakfast cereal

Day 5: muffin and coffee

Day 6: fresh fruit

Day 7: fresh vegetables

Day 1: Scrambled eggs alone left me feeling icky, like a lump in my stomache, but I wasn't quite full, so I added 2 pieces of whole grain toast to the equation which made me feel better. 2 hrs later I was feeling fine. 3 hrs later needed a snack

Day 2: Oatmeal (Hot multigrain cereal) Fills me up making me feel a bit bloated at first, but I'm hungry again 2 hours later.

Day 3: Muffin & coffee. Try#1 Does the trick for about four hours, but then I crash in the afternoon. Try#2: Yikes major tummy ache

Day 4: _Boxed breakfast cereal w/ soymilk._ _____

_____

_____

_____

Day 5: _____

_____

_____

_____

Day 6: _____

_____

_____

_____

Day 7: _____

_____

_____

_____

When you have the knack, you can expand the experiment to include your whole daily intake, exploring how different foods and liquids affect you. For example, for one week, make a point of drinking more water during the day, or eating more leafy greens or meat. Notice how your body feels, how each change of diet affects your mood.

2. Metabolic Type Test

Go to www.alkalizeforhealth.net/Lmetabolictype.htm and take a test to find your metabolic type. You can use this information, along with listening to your body's messages and keeping a Food-Mood Journal, to create awareness about the foods that are easy for you to digest.

What is your metabolic type?

_____

How is this information going to influence the choices you make around food and exercise?

_____

_____

_____

_____

3. Mindful Eating

The best way to bring more awareness and understanding to your eating habits is to slow everything down. Take time selecting your food and choosing the place where you will eat it. Make a little ritual before you begin, pressing the palms of your hands together in a namaste, saying a prayer or giving thanks. Eat one spoonful at a time. Do not take another bite until the one in your mouth has been chewed and swallowed. Chew slowly. See if you can chew your food for 30 seconds per mouthful, noticing how saliva builds in your mouth as the food is pulped by the grinding movement of your teeth. Notice how the flavors of food are released as you chew. Take time to appreciate their subtle qualities. At the end of your meal, use another small ritual to bring it to a close. Write down your experiences.

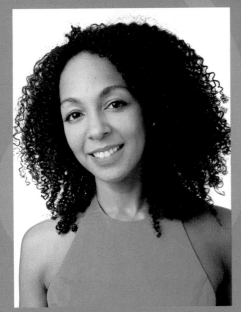

I have an MBA from Harvard Business School and spent seven years working at MTV Networks. I rose very quickly to be one of the youngest vice presidents there, and my earnings were in the top 1% of the country. I was having fun, but I wasn't very balanced. I pushed my body to the brink, ended up in the hospital and almost died from a stress-induced ulcerated digestive system, which was diagnosed as Crohn's disease.

The experience of almost dying in the hospital changed my perspective on everything. A couple of years afterwards, I decided to leave my job to open one of the first yoga studios in Harlem, the Ta Yoga House. People thought I had lost my mind, but I was in the process of finding myself. I was on a quest to create a more sustainable, health-supportive lifestyle. That's when I found Integrative Nutrition. It put me in touch with other like-minded people looking to change their lives. Being in a community full of change agents is a powerful force, and I was guided closer to my purpose.

In school I deepened my knowledge about cooking, digestion, the importance of stress management, breathing, meditation and food therapies. I started to incorporate what I learned into the Ta Yoga offerings, in the form of cooking classes and holistic health workshops.

One day during the school year the brand "Power Living" came to me. It was about healthy and successful living. I went full force in developing Power Living Enterprises, Inc. During the process, I converted Ta Yoga into an organization for the community, and began to focus more of my attention on building Power Living as a for-profit brand. We offer lifestyle and success coaching, personal development training programs for corporations and motivational products.

Today I am a sought-after motivational speaker and have spoken to thousands of people at events, ranging from the Harvard Business School Women's Alumnae Association and Essence Work & Wealth Seminar to Elmhurst Hospital and Abyssinian Baptist Church. I have also been featured in media around the world, from *O: The Oprah Magazine* and *Yoga Journal* to NBC's *Today in New York* and ARD TV in Germany. I'm getting the message of Power Living out there to larger and larger audiences. I am writing a book, and we are developing a television show. I am melding my skills from my years in media, holistic health and yoga to help people on a broader basis.

On a personal level, I follow my own principles. Most people with Crohn's get very sick, but I do not have any digestive symptoms at all. This is amazing. As in hatha yoga, life is a balance between effort and ease. I now know when to push hard and when to ease up. I take time to pause and play. I am Power Living! Thank you Integrative Nutrition for being a part of my transformation.

Teresa Kay-Aba Kennedy
New York, NY
Graduate 2003
www.power-living.com

chapter 3

When it comes to diet,
one size definitely doesn't fit all.

Christiane Northrup, MD

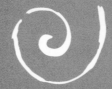

dietary theory

I HAVE ALWAYS BEEN INTERESTED IN food. It was exciting to go shopping with my mother, to pick things off the shelf and to put them all away when we got home. Then she would let me help with the cooking. When I grew up, my academic education focused on psychology and counseling, but my passion for food never left. In fact, it grew as I noticed the strong relationship between my clients' diets and their openness to new ideas and change.

Soon I developed an interest in natural foods, and began exploring macrobiotics. I studied extensively with Michio and Aveline Kushi, some of the chief students of George Ohsawa, the man who created macrobiotics as it is known today.

Macrobiotics has been a fruitful source of nutritional principles for many people, including Paul Pitchford, Dr. Dean Ornish and Dr. Christiane Northrup. My creation of our school evolved out of this Japanese-based theory, and I'd like to share a few stories to illustrate why macrobiotics attracted me, and why I later felt the need to expand to a wider vision.

Michio and Aveline were known for their finely tuned taste buds and skill in judging how food was prepared by its taste alone. They would go to a meal and intuitively know who at the table had prepared each dish and what his or her thoughts and feelings were. They knew so much about a person by just tasting his or her food. One day Vince decided he was going to test their abilities, and put all kinds of crazy energy into a dish he was preparing. When it came time to taste the food, Michio, with studied Japanese politeness, commented, "This is good, but very strange." Then, at the end of the meal, he turned to my colleague and said calmly, "Maybe you need a doctor."

On another occasion, I was preparing a meal for 10 people as part of my certification exam at the

Kushi Institute, and it was suddenly announced that Michio had returned to the U.S. from a visit to Japan and would be coming for dinner, along with his entourage of 10 extra people. This was an hour before mealtime. Since there was no way I had time to prepare more food, I decided to add more soba noodles to the soba dish and more water to the soup. This way, I thought, things would be more or less okay for my exam.

When Michio and Aveline arrived, they inspected the food, admired its appearance and offered a prayer. Everyone sat down and began to eat. There was utter silence in the room as we awaited their verdict. Michio tasted it and said, "You add water to the soup at the end of its cooking." At that moment it felt as if only he and I were in the room, and like a young student trying to avoid punishment for cheating in class, I said, "No." Then I realized how dumb this behavior was and I confessed, explaining my concern and thought process about how to feed 20 people.

My embarrassment was surpassed by my being truly impressed that someone could know, just through taste, that water had been added to a soup towards the end of its preparation. I realized the depth of Michio's understanding and the levels of subtlety that exist in cooking and consuming food. At that moment, he inspired me to commit my life to the development of this kind of understanding. I grasped the idea of using my body as a walking, talking laboratory in which I could conduct a vast array of experiments, seeking optimum health.

For a while macrobiotics supplied all the answers for me. Like many dietary theories, it promised amazing results for those who followed its complex rules, but there were some issues that wouldn't go away. It's common knowledge to people who study at the Kushi Institute and attend macrobiotic conferences that many macrobiotic teachers smoke cigarettes, drink alcohol and enjoyed eating donuts on a regular basis. This seemed odd to me since the macrobiotic diet is so rigid in its forbidding tomatoes, potatoes, oranges, garlic and many other everyday foods. Over time, these contradictions were helpful because they freed me from becoming a true believer and sent me on a quest to gather a broader base of knowledge and information.

I was assisted in this quest by my experience living at Kripalu, the largest residential yoga center in the U.S. I was amazed and inspired that they taught so many different types of yoga. Through participating in that process, I began to see the beauty and wisdom of assimilating all the types of yoga from different kinds of teachers, instead of having to chose one right away. I could see the implications as far as diet programs were concerned. If I could apply the same principle of acceptance to nutrition, how wonderful that would be! I decided to develop a new kind of nutrition school, one that would teach the best of every diet system and help people sort out for themselves which one to choose and follow.

I was eager for the new adventure ahead of me and the challenge of presenting different theories. Most people in nutrition believe that their theory is the right one and that everyone else's theory is wrong. They see the emergence of new information as competition and attempt to dismiss other diet plans as fad diets.

My approach is the opposite. Based on my own experiences with the power of integrating the teachings of various schools of thought, I am thrilled when new dietary theories emerge. I am fascinated by the continued reaching towards the discovery of what is true and what will help us live happier, healthier lives. When a new theory appears, I read about it, research it, try to understand where its creators are coming from, and then add their wisdom to the school's repertoire. Something in me says, "Great! Another ray of light is being shed on our crazy eating habits. Here's one more researcher who understands the link between nutrition and health, and has taken time and energy to develop a new perspective."

Our school teaches all the different dietary theories, covering the pros and cons of each. And the interesting thing is they all work. They all don't work, too, but I'll come to that in a moment. Why do all diets work? Because when people decide to go on a diet, they have already realized that what they are eating is not working for them and it's time for a change. People become conscious about their self-destructive eating habits. Maybe it's after the Christmas/New Year break and they have put on five pounds, they feel bad, and the threat of obesity is staring them in the face. The scale in the bathroom is groaning, their clothes just went up a size, and now they want to be more aware of their food habits. They vow to cut out binging, eat more veggies, exercise regularly, and drink more water instead of coffee and alcohol.

In this situation, whatever diet they choose is going to work because they are moving away from a chaotic, disordered way of eating to an ordered way of eating. They are going to stop eating chemicalized artificial junk food, and they are going to get better. The general rule is that any attention to diet is better than none. Diet theorists miss this because they want to attribute success to their unique approach.

In reality, all diet programs contain elements of truth. When we talk about various diets in class, including programs ranging from raw foods to Atkins, there are always students who swear that a particular diet really helped them. The extent to which people can benefit from specific diets is amazing. This is yet another reminder to appreciate the extent to which we, as a species, are so diverse and unique.

It is my belief that when a diet is successful there may be a placebo effect at work as well. This is not often discussed in the field of nutrition. Many studies have been done over the years that illustrate the power of suggestion. When a group of patients all suffering from the same ailment are given sugar pills and told the pills represent a breakthrough treatment, a significant percentage of the patients will recover simply by taking the sugar pills. It's the same with diets. Many of them work as much because of this self-hypnosis factor as any intrinsic value in the program itself.

The truth is that most people will lose weight on any given diet program for a limited period of time only, and then revert to a less disciplined way of eating. Why? Because most diet books instruct people to eat a narrow band of recommended food. People follow the program with all good intentions, slowly narrowing their list of acceptable foods, squeezing their eyes shut while scurrying past a Dunkin' Donuts or Starbucks in a determined effort not to stray from the chosen path. Sooner or later, the craving for what is missing becomes too great, their determination fades and they fall off the wagon. This is not because they are weak, ignorant or lack willpower, but because humans are omnivorous creatures with roving appetites; we love to experiment with food. So it is that as all diets work, they don't work too.

I know the power of the human appetite from personal experience. During the stage of my life when I was more or less vegetarian, I tried to avoid animal foods as much as possible. Eventually my craving for meat grew so strong that late one evening I found my car pulling into a fast food drive-through. I saw myself ordering a burger with extra, extra vegetables and parking on a deserted street to wolf down the forbidden food. I had never experienced such exhilaration. I felt so good and so bad simultaneously. My covert behavior continued for many years until I could come to a deeper, clearer understanding of a balanced way of eating.

This understanding was a result of listening to my own body and studying any and every dietary theory I could, as I have described. Following is a description of several of these theories, including the pros and cons of each.

• • • Macrobiotics • • •

The modern macrobiotic movement began with George Ohsawa, a Japanese dietary innovator who lived in the first half of the 20th century, and combined Eastern philosophy with food and medicine. Macrobiotics uses a modified version of the ancient concept of yin-yang, which points to an underlying order in the universe based on a dynamic, ever-changing balance between two apparently opposite yet complementary principles. Yang embodies qualities like masculine, hard, strong, active, tight and contractive. Yin embodies the feminine, soft, yielding, passive, receptive, loose and expansive. The dance between these two universal energies includes not only men and women, yang foods and yin foods, but day and night, winter and summer, good and bad, sweet and salty; it goes on and on.

Originally, I wasn't interested in the dietary aspect of macrobiotics. I was inspired by the simple, ancient wisdom of the yin-yang philosophy and the dance of opposites. How could anyone overlook such a simple and self-evident system of universal dynamics? As I studied further, I learned that Ohsawa's key to good health is to maintain yin-yang balance by following a traditional, grain-based diet. He taught there is only one basic human disease: living out of balance. He asserted that the age-old concept of grains as the principal food in diet, a sacred food in virtually every traditional society, had largely vanished from the West. He was also the first to introduce brown rice and soy products as staple foods in Europe and America.

When I teach about the history of macrobiotics, I explain how it originated in an enclosed Japanese island culture with limited food resources, where they were obliged to eat the same foods—rice, local vegetables, fish and seaweed—over and over again. They did not have dairy or much animal meat. To keep their meals appetizing, they developed different ways to cook the same food, often based on the season of year. They cooked the exact same food one way in winter and another way in summer. Through this practice, they developed a healthy way of eating that greatly impressed Western doctors because there was no cholesterol problem and much less heart disease in Japan. I should mention that the traditional Japanese diet relies heavily on salt for flavoring. Miso soup, for example, is very salty, as are soy sauce and umeboshi plums. Unfortunately, as a result of this overabundance of salt, stomach cancer is a significant problem among the Japanese.

When I first encountered macrobiotics, eating seasonal, locally grown, organic produce and traditional foods was new and exciting. I was also attracted by lifestyle-improving suggestions like the use of a hot towel scrub (I'll describe this in chapter 7). Another suggestion I appreciated was to sing a happy song every day. It really surprised me. A singing diet? Unbelievable! But when I did it, I noticed I felt better, and this opened my mind to the concept of being nourished on different levels, not only physically, but also mentally, emotionally and spiritually.

Other macrobiotic suggestions include keeping your home simple, neat and clean, wearing more cotton clothes and less synthetic fibers, maintaining a sense of humor, allowing time for prayer and meditation, avoiding excessive jewelry or chemicalized perfume, and keeping green plants in the home. There is also a recommendation to be on good terms with all people.

For several years I maintained what I would call a vegan macrobiotic diet—meaning no dairy, meat, honey or eggs. I did eat fish about once a month. I became very healthy and strong, and any time I went for a checkup all my numbers would be right down the center. Gradually, however, I began to notice the downside of this way of eating. Even though macrobiotics advises people to eat the traditional diet of their ancestors, most macrobiotic teachings, books and sections in natural food stores strongly emphasize Japanese foods. This wasn't too big a problem when I started my nutrition school in Toronto, but when I moved to New York I found I was dealing with a much more diverse clientele, with students who had to go home after class and feed Puerto Rican, African American and Jewish families. To try and impose a Japanese diet on such people is practically an invitation to break up their families. Moreover, the task of preparing complex macrobiotic recipes for New York's singles or working moms was adding unnecessary stress to their already crowded daily schedule.

The saltiness of the diet is another issue. Condiments and flavoring other than salt are considered less helpful to macrobiotic cooking. It rarely incorporates herbs and spices, and sugar is abhorred, so salt is added to everything. Every medical student and health practitioner knows that too much salt can lead to hypertension—feeling increasingly tense—accompanied by rising blood pressure, and the first thing a doctor recommends if a patient has high blood pressure is they cut out salt.

The really difficult part of the macrobiotic diet is the suggestion to drink only when thirsty. There is a scientific understanding that the body doesn't normally get thirsty enough to let you know when you are dehydrated, a kind of neurological time lag. Our body needs water, but our brain doesn't get the message, so we don't feel the urge to drink until dehydration has already happened. I spent five years on a macrobiotic diet, and I never thought I was thirsty. My body was used to a very low level of water.

Having too much salt and not enough water are both independently problematic for the body, but to combine the two is a recipe for disaster. Paul Pitchford, author of *Healing with Whole Foods: Asian Traditions and Modern Nutrition*, told me the story of a woman who decided to include a lot of miso (fermented soy beans) in her diet because she felt it was high in protein and easy for her body to assimilate. She also followed the macrobiotic principle of not drinking much water, and as a result became dehydrated, weak and emaciated. One day she went hiking with a companion and came to an outlook point at the top of a cliff where they could see a waterfall. She exclaimed to her friend, "Look at the water! It's so beautiful!" Walking towards the water, she fell off the edge of the cliff and died. In a way, she died of thirst. This tragic story shows that even though your head can convince your body to obey a diet for a while, your body will reach a certain point and reassert itself.

It's amazing how people can get carried away with their beliefs, confusing food with religious fervor, and macrobiotics certainly has its share of fanatics. To such people I want to say, "It's just a diet. It doesn't matter that much. You will not go to hell for drinking too much water."

● ● ● Ayurveda ● ● ●

The ancient Indian healing system called Ayurveda, which translates to "the science of life" in Sanskrit, was developed at least 3,000 years ago. In recent times, Ayurvedic medicine and its accompanying herbal remedies has become increasingly popular in the U.S. and Europe. Ayurveda recognizes that all life—

whether it be human, plant or animal—must live in harmony with nature in order to survive. Creating optimal health and balance begins by adopting the concept of "food as medicine."

In Ayurveda, proper diet is coupled with the three seasons. The late fall harvest is rich in nuts and grains—all warming and insulating to combat the cold, dry extremes of the coming winter. Meat is eaten more at this time as well. In the summer, when it becomes hot, the naturally occurring harvest is rich in cooling fruits and vegetables. Eating those in-season fruits and vegetables in abundance naturally wards off the accumulated heat of summer. In the wet, rainy and congested spring, the naturally occurring harvest is rich in dry, low fat and astringent roots, sprouts, grapefruits and berries. These foods help to decrease the seasonal tendency to make mucus, and fight against allergies, colds and weight gain. Cultures that are still connected to the local farmer practice these universal principles of Ayurveda by naturally changing their diets with the rhythm of the seasons.

Nature is made up of five elements: space, air, fire, water and earth. As nature materializes itself, these five elements combine to create the three basic fundamental principles in nature, called doshas. Space and air combine to form the principle called vata. Fire and water combine to form the principle called pitta. And earth and water combine to form kapha. These principles are used to categorize body type. Thus, there are three seasons, three primary harvests and three body types.

If this system intrigues you, I encourage you study it further. If you find the right practitioner, it can be an incredible tool for creating health and balance. However, be aware that the west has simplified this very ancient system of medicine. We have created a very marketable version of Ayurveda: know your

vata

The qualities of vata as seen in nature are cold, dry, rough and constantly moving. Winter is the season in which vata predominates. During this time of year it is cold, our skin gets dry, precipitation becomes cold and dry in the form of snow, and the wind blows without restriction as the trees are without leaves.

The vata body type is what we imagine when we think of our contemporary notion of beauty: thin-boned, tall and skinny, or short, slim and petite. Vatas have sharp minds and a tendency to worry; they are light sleepers and have nervous dispositions. These people usually have a fast metabolism, experience difficulty gaining weight, and are characteristically weak in their intestines, suffering from poor absorption of nutrients. As the squirrel needs nuts in the winter and as the natural harvest is rich in warm, heavy foods, so the wintry vata requires highly nutritious food, with an abundance of cooked vegetables and whole grains to promote healthy assimilation and bowel function. They benefit from eating small amounts of animal food, but must be careful not to overdo it. Fish and low fat meats are usually best.

Vatas need regular exercise to release nervous tension. They do best with more meditative, gentle and calming practices such as yoga.

pitta

During the summer months, the environment accumulates heat. This property of fire or heat is called pitta.

Pitta body types embody the qualities of fire. This body type is physically oriented, with more muscle and a fiery temperament. Pitta people usually have yellow- or reddish-colored skin that is sensitive to rashes. They often sweat profusely, and are easily irritated. Their bodies and temperaments both tend to be hot. For the most part, they have a very strong and athletic constitution.

Pittas tend to be leaders and are well organized, intelligent and charismatic. They are usually emotional, competitive, passionate and in need of a good eight hours' sleep per night to rest and cool off. They have enormous appetites for food and life experience, and can become gluttons if not careful. Their weakest physical points are their liver, heart and stomach.

Pittas benefit from seeking balance in eating, avoiding hot spices and too much animal food, emphasizing sweet vegetables like squash and pumpkin, and whole grains like barley and oats. Most importantly, pitas must avoid excess and include regular exercise in their daily schedule.

kapha

Spring, which is the kapha season, is a very wet and heavy time of year. It is allergy season, the rainy season, full of heavy mud and potential congestion.

Influenced by the qualities of springtime, those with kapha body types are big-boned, full-bodied and physically strong, and tend toward weight gain. Their solid skeletons protect them from osteoporosis. Skin color is pale and cool, and eyes large and often dark. They are frequently easygoing, slow, methodical types, with balanced, peaceful temperaments. Kapha types radiate competence, even when they are quiet or shy.

Kaphas have a slow metabolism and strong intestines, and the ease with which they assimilate nutrients means that they don't have to eat much to stay in good health. In fact, they should avoid overeating because their main health concern is the danger of obesity. The heart is their weakest organ.

Kaphas should eat lots of vegetables and light foods, including a wide range of grains. Their primary animal food should be eggs. All spices are good for kaphas, but they need to restrict intake of oil as much as possible. Regular, nonstrenuous physical exercise, like taking a stroll in the park, suits them best.

body type and know thyself. But there is more to it than that. While understanding one's body type is important, it is by no means the core of Ayurveda. In India, Ayurvedic doctors usually do not tell a patient their body type. Instead, they are concerned about the imbalance of the patient. The critical information is our susceptibility to imbalance. With this information we can employ preventative techniques to avoid disease and maintain good health.

For people with a strong yoga practice, Ayurveda can be the perfect diet because its philosophy meshes so well with yoga. But for many westerners looking for a quick fix, Ayurveda can be confusing. Many books and practitioners guide people to an Indian based cuisine using recipes and ingredients unfamiliar to the western palate. For a single person, this can be fun and new and experimental, but for families this can create chaos, as mom tries yet another new food experiment. Then there is also the challenge of new words and concepts and finally the problem of dealing with a home situation where family members require different diets, because they have a different body types. Our greatest lesson from Ayurveda is to learn from nature, eat in harmony with the seasons and live a life of balance.

• • • 5 Element Theory • • •

Based on ancient Chinese philosophy, the 5 Element Theory relates all energy and substance to the elements—fire, earth, metal (or air), water and wood. Each element is associated with one of the directions of the compass and one of the seasons, including Indian summer as the fifth season. One element gives birth to the next and nourishes it through the flow of energy. This is the creation cycle. Wood creates fire, which creates earth, which creates metal, which creates water, which creates wood. The other cycle is the destruction cycle, whereby wood injures earth, fire destroys metal, earth controls water, metal attacks wood and water injures fire.

Wood represents the morning as the time of day, and spring as the season. It is associated with the organs of the liver and the gallbladder and the emotions of impatience and anger. The wood vegetables are artichoke, broccoli, carrot, string beans, sprouts, parsley and leafy greens. The effect of wood on the body is purification.

The fire time of day is noon, the season is summer and the related organs are the heart and small intestine. The related emotion is joy. Fire vegetables are asparagus, brussels sprout, beet, chive, dandelion, scallion and tomato. Coffee and tobacco are also fiery. Fire creates circulation in the body.

Afternoon and Indian summer are associated with the earth element. The stomach and pancreas are the associated organs, and sympathy and worry are the correlated emotions. Chard, collards, parsnips, spinach, squash and sweet potato are the earth vegetables. The taste of earth is sweet, and other common earth substances are carob, honey, maple syrup and sugar. The related bodily function of earth is digestion.

Metal is associated with the evening, autumn, the lungs and grief. Cabbage, cauliflower, celery, cucumber, daikon and radish are the metal vegetables. Peppermint, spirulina, tofu and tempeh also belong to the metal family, along with respiration as the bodily function.

Water is linked with night, winter, kidneys and the bladder. The emotion is fear. Beets, burdock, sea vegetables and kale are water vegetables. Miso, salt and tamari are also water foods. Elimination is the bodily function.

In this theory, the way you cook changes the energy of your food. Stir-frying and deep frying give food wood energy, grilling and barbequing give food fire energy, boiling gives food water energy, baking gives food metal energy and steaming gives food earth energy.

People who know which foods, seasons, emotions and bodily functions are associated with which element are masters of balance. Say, for example, it's the middle of winter and you are feeling constipated and tight. According to the 5 Element Theory it's the water time of year, so increasing sea vegetables and drinking more water could help. Or say that you are craving coffee and cigarettes, which both belong to the fire element. You could look at those cravings and ask yourself, "Where else can I add fire, passion and joy into my life?" You could also increase the fire vegetables and bitter taste in your diet. Chances are your craving for coffee and cigarettes would subside.

If you are interested in exploring this theory further, it can be helpful to get a poster with the elements and components of each element clearly listed and to create a food journal, writing down what you eat ever day for breakfast, lunch and dinner, and recording how much food you eat from each element. This will help you see your natural tendencies and find balance. For instance, if you notice that you are eating mostly earth foods, it may help to increase wood foods because wood holds down the earth.

• • • High Carbohydrate Diets • • •

I would pinpoint 1972 as the beginning of the trend towards high carbohydrate diets in America, with the publication of a book titled *Diet for a Small Planet* by Frances Moore Lappé. This book eventually sold more than 3 million copies worldwide. Lappé asserted that it is human practices, not natural disasters that cause worldwide hunger. Food scarcity results when grain, rich in nutrients and capable of supporting vast populations, is fed to livestock to produce meat, which yields only a fraction of those nutrients. Lappé presented a theory of how traditional cultures stay healthy by mixing certain kinds of vegetable proteins together. The timing of her book coincided with an American hippie subculture that was turning its back on fast food and embracing natural foods, macrobiotics, Indian-style vegetarianism and a grain-based diet as part of a general "back to the land" movement.

Then came Nathan Pritikin, who studied indigenous cultures around the world and noted they did not have the types of chronic disease suffered by people in developed countries. He attributed their health to a low fat diet with lots of carbohydrates. Based on these insights, he created the Pritikin Longevity Center in 1976. In 1980 he co-authored a best-selling book, *The Pritikin Program for Diet and Exercise*, in which he advocated a low fat, low protein diet, with most of its nutrition coming from complex carbohydrates. Recommended foods included fresh and cooked fruits and vegetables, whole grains, bread, pasta, and small amounts of lean meat, fish and poultry. He also encouraged daily regimens of aerobic exercise.

In 1977 George McGovern, the director of the Food for Peace program under John F. Kennedy, headed the U.S. Senate Select Committee on Nutrition and Human Needs, which boosted the movement towards vegetable and grain-based diets. This was unwelcome news for the meat and dairy industries. Six years later, in 1983, Dr. John McDougall attracted public attention by offering a vegan diet of high carbohydrate, low protein foods, and then in 1993 Dr. Dean Ornish published the best-selling book titled *Eat More, Weigh Less*. The title of Ornish's book was helpful because it shattered the commonly held notion that losing weight requires starvation. To actually eat more and still shed pounds was a truly revolutionary idea. Ornish embraced macrobiotics, but had the entrepreneurial savvy to drop the Japanese element and yin-yang philosophy, as well as the seaweed and miso. He stuck with the system's basic dietary principles.

In 1988 the U.S. Surgeon General, in conjunction with the American Medical Association, conducted a study of various weight loss plans. The study showed that two-thirds of people on those plans gained all their weight back in one year, while 97% regained all their weight within five years. A few years later, Ornish showed that under his plan, patients lost 24 pounds in the first year and kept more than half the weight off for five years, attributing much of his success to the fact that his patients could eat more food, thereby avoiding hunger pangs and cravings normally associated with dieting.

The next thing Ornish did was approach insurance companies like Blue Cross Blue Shield, pointing out how much money they could save on payouts for heart bypass surgery if they instead paid for their clients to participate in his program. In response, the companies put 300 people on his program and saved millions of dollars for themselves. The Ornish program for reversing heart disease is now accepted by insurance companies as a deductible expense. This is a huge breakthrough for the nutrition world. The Ornish program recommends a diet largely of grains and vegetables, with a formula of 10% fat, 20% protein and 70% carbohydrates. He also recommends yoga, meditation and developing a loving heart—hugging is healthy—to keep the arteries clean and clear.

One more person I should mention here is Dr. Anne Louise Gittleman, former head nutritionist at the Pritikin Center, who was the first to see the problem side of a low fat, high carbohydrate diet. She observed that Eskimos eat a diet of 70% fat and have no heart disease, and from this starting point she was able to distinguish between bad fats—such as saturated fats in dairy products and trans fats in processed foods like potato chips and margarine—and good fats that help keep people healthy—like olive oil, avocado, omega 3, omega 6 and oils from seeds and nuts. In fact, as later research has shown, absence of these good fats may create just the kind of heart disease dangers that low fat diets are trying to avoid because they prevent the accumulation of cholesterol and triglycerides in our arteries. Omega 3 fatty acids, found predominantly in fish oil, are especially effective at scavenging and removing these unwanted elements.

Gittleman also pointed out that the average American does not know the difference between healthy and unhealthy carbohydrates. The experts might be talking about the need to eat brown rice, millet, quinoa, corn, whole grain breads, vegetables and beans, but most Americans have no idea what these foods are, or where to buy them. As a result, they eat more refined wheat products, more bread, pasta and pizza, and this plays havoc with people's blood sugar levels. In addition, Gittleman warned about the dangers caused by gluten in wheat, which acts like a kind of glue in the body and can cause allergies, brain fog, candida and mineral deficiencies. Gittleman's contribution to understanding the subtleties and implications of this diet is significant.

As a teacher of nutrition, I can tell you that one of the biggest challenges facing people on high carbohydrate diets is monotony and boredom. Eating meals consisting largely of grains and veggies may be great for the body's health, but it can be a very frustrating experience for the palate. One thing you must learn if you are going to make a high carbohydrate diet work for you is how to make simple food taste delicious. I'll explain this further in chapter 9.

People love eating protein. It makes us feel stronger, more alert and more aggressive. It increases our sense of power and confidence, two of the most highly prized qualities in our contemporary culture, which is part of the reason high protein diets are so popular today. Another reason high protein diets are flourishing right now is because they can cause weight loss, sometimes of significant proportion.

A lot of people who embrace high protein diets follow the program prescribed by Dr. Robert Atkins, who began his work in 1972 with the publication of *Dr. Atkins' Diet Revolution*, and who died in 2003, at the age of 73. The title of a recently released biography about Atkins, *The True Story of the Man Behind the War on Carbohydrates*, amply describes his life's mission. Atkins' supporters claim that, under his plan, you can "eat delicious meals you love, never count calories, enjoy a cheeseburger when you're hungry, see amazing results in 14 days, reach your ideal weight and stay there." They also say you can eat all the meat and all the fat you want. With such a generous range of permitted foods, how could anyone not want to go on such a program?

Atkins and similar high protein programs cause weight loss by depriving the body of the carbohydrates that our digestive system routinely converts into sugar, its preferred fuel. Once the body recognizes that it is not getting carbohydrates, it will burn protein for a few days in their place. But thousands of years of evolutionary experience as hunter-gatherers has taught us that burning protein is not a good idea because protein is our primary muscle constituent. Without muscle we have no strength to hunt for food. Therefore, burning protein is counterproductive to survival, so the body doesn't like to do it, and won't do it for very long.

Once the carbohydrate stores are burned, and we've burned protein for a few days, our body says, "It's time to start burning fat." At this point, our brain says, "No, I don't like this," because it prefers only carbohydrates as a fuel source. So our liver performs a little chemical magic and converts fat into ketones, a substance which the brain can burn. Now our body is in a state of ketosis, burning fat and losing weight, just the way we want.

This is not the only way high protein diets cause weight loss. During the first few days on the program the body loses a lot of water, which accounts for much of the lost weight at the outset. This initial weight loss encourages us to continue. High protein diets also reduce hunger, which means we eat less. Atkins is popular because it's a fast way to lose weight while eating bacon, chicken and pork, therefore avoiding starvation. But not many of us can sustain this way of eating for a long period of time. We all know someone who has been on Atkins, but do you know anyone who has stayed on it? People go on the diet, lose weight, tell their friends about it, and by the time their friends have bought the book, they are off the diet and have gained the weight back. This cycle is how Atkins has become so popular.

The Atkins approach could benefit many vegetarian-type people. Vegetarians often suffer from extreme ups and downs with their blood sugar levels. This simply doesn't happen to those on the Atkins program. When a vegetarian goes on Atkins, the pancreas gets to rest because their sugar consumption decreases while protein intake increases. People who suffer from candida or diabetes, two illnesses that are aggravated by too much sugar consumption, can sometimes benefit from this way of eating for a short time.

Atkins Nutritionals Inc., a fast-growing international enterprise that owns the Atkins trademark and markets a wide range of products related to the diet, recently came out with its own USDA-style food guide pyramid. The Atkins pyramid puts protein at the base as the foundational structure of the diet, eliminates refined grains—something the government hasn't yet had the courage to do—and warns against the health hazards of sugar and trans fat. It retains fruits and vegetables, selecting only those vegetables low in sugar content, not including squash, onions or carrots. Contrary to the USDA guidelines, it emphasizes the importance of fats.

The downside to Atkins and other high protein diets is that too much animal protein may lead to complications in the body, especially heart disease and cancer. This danger does not apply to everybody, but animal meat is full of saturated fats that can spike blood cholesterol levels, has no fiber to aid digestion and is low in many essential plant-based nutrients, such as antioxidants, carotenoids and phytochemicals. In addition, there is increasing concern about tainted meat, mad cow disease, and the presence of hormones and antibiotics in factory-farmed meat. If you decide to go on the Atkins diet, you should eat organic animal food as much as possible.

Another problem is that this program doesn't really distinguish between eating beef, fish, chicken or eggs. To Atkins, a protein is a protein is a protein, whereas in reality, each of these has a completely different quality and impact on the body, as I discussed in chapter 2.

Further, the body is meant to maintain a balance between the acidic and the alkaline. Protein is a very acidic substance. If you eat a lot of it, your body will seek to create a more alkaline environment in your stomach. It does this by leaching calcium from your bones and teeth, and this may contribute to bone loss and osteoporosis.

People also say these diets are taxing for the kidneys, create constipation, depression, bad breath and body odors. At the beginning of each year at our school, I ask the new students about the kinds of diets they've attempted, and how they felt while they were on them. When asking about high protein programs, these are some of the responses I've received:

"I felt very tight," one woman said. "The diet created a lot of tension in me. It was as if my entire body felt squeezed."

Another person said, "The more protein I ate, the more aggressive and anxious I became. After a while, I didn't recognize myself."

"Constipated," said one, succinctly. "I had to take laxatives. I felt like my bowels shut down."

"I was always craving carbs, anything—a bagel, bread, pastries," a woman told me. "Every time I walked past the bakery aisle in my supermarket or the donut shop near my apartment I had to resist running in and eating whole trays of baked goods. I couldn't wait to lose the weight so I could stop eating that way."

"I couldn't stand eating all that meat, cheese and fat," one man said. "It made me feel greasy."

Next, I ask, "But did these high protein diets cause weight loss?"

"Yes!" Everyone consistently replies.

"Were you able to keep that weight off?"

"No!"

• • • The Zone Diet • • •

The Zone Diet was developed by Dr. Barry Sears, author of the best-seller *Enter the Zone*, and is based on over 15 years of his research in the field of bio-nutrition. It is sometimes called a high protein diet, but is less extreme than Atkins and aims at decreasing weight without hunger pangs. The diet's primary aim, as the name suggests, is to keep you in "the zone," an expression drawn from the world of sports and used to describe an almost mystical state of heightened awareness and relaxed intensity in which athletes suddenly find themselves producing their best performance without effort. Clearly, no diet can guarantee access to such an intense experience, but the Zone Diet does promise to help you feel good. The goal is to get so that you are not feeling overly tense or anxious, not depressed or lethargic, not thinking about food, not overeating and not starving. Your energy level is optimal for normal day-to-day living.

The Zone offers a specific meal plan based on each person's gender, activity level and amount of body fat. It's called "the 40-30-30 diet" because you get 40% of your calories from carbohydrates, 30% from protein and 30% from fat. This contrasts sharply with the accepted nutritional standard of 65-15-20. All meals and snacks follow the 40-30-30 ratio on the grounds that the more you give your body 40-30-30, the more it gets accustomed to processing this food combination, and the sooner your body will settle into a specific metabolic state leading to weight loss. Sears takes the view that your body is a machine and it has no political or philosophical views on vegetarianism, animal rights or food politics. You just give it the right-formula fuel to burn and it will run at optimum capacity, not wasting energy digesting excess food.

One of the goals of the Zone is to avoid peaks and valleys in blood sugar levels, and a recommendation that I find effective is to eat a meal within one hour after waking because that's when your blood sugar is lowest. The Zone persuades people to eat more fruits and vegetables, and reduce bread, pasta and white grains. It is big on drinking water, which I agree with wholeheartedly. I also like the Zone's relaxed attitude about mistakes: no big deal if you fall off the diet since you are only one meal away from getting back on track. Another aspect of the Zone Diet that I like is its direction to eat five times a day, three meals and two snacks. Never allow more than five hours to pass without eating, and it's okay to eat when you are not hungry. If you continue eating proper ratio meals and snacks, you'll never feel hungry or overly stuffed; you will always be in the Zone, with normal blood sugar levels throughout the day and night. People on the diet say to me, "Yes, this is great, I am never hungry, always in the Zone, and it works!"

According to Zone theory, your stomach doesn't distinguish between a carrot and a candy bar. So a carb is a carb is a carb, and high carbohydrate foods need to be avoided. To me, this is ridiculous. A carrot is made naturally with sun, wind and earth energy, whereas a candy bar is a manufactured, artificial product. Your body knows the difference and will respond accordingly. Similarly, the Zone makes no distinction between sources of protein and so, like Atkins, the risk of diseases caused by animal foods is present. Another downside is that it's hard to make every meal 40-30-30. Unless you are a scientist, making each meal perfectly balanced is virtually impossible.

It's difficult to be on a Zone diet and be a vegetarian because of the diet's strong emphasis on eating protein. In response, the Zone people came out with what they call Soy Zone, recommending more soy products. But many people are allergic to soy or have difficulty digesting it in big quantities.

Critics of the Zone often argue that weight loss on this program comes from restricting calories and not from any bio-chemical magic induced by the 40-30-30 formula. They also assert that, contrary to Sears' claims, athletic performance may be impaired by reducing carbohydrates.

South Beach is southern Florida's most fashionable beach and a showcase of human bodies that have been carefully groomed, styled and shaped—often with help from cosmetic surgery—to display maximum fitness, health and beauty. When South Beach's own Dr. Arthur Agatston, a cardiologist, developed a diet for his heart patients and saw the dramatic weight-loss results, he published it as a way to help people walk the Florida sands in front of their peers without shame or embarrassment.

At first glance, this diet may not seem very different from other high protein, low carbohydrate weight loss plans. But South Beach focuses more on the type and quality of carbohydrates consumed, using the glycemic index to differentiate. The glycemic index shows how quickly a particular food makes your blood sugar rise, a measuring system that is used in nutritional management of diabetes. "This new way of eating allows you to live contently without eating bad carbohydrates and fats," asserts the South Beach program. "In contrast, when a person eats poor quality carbohydrates and fats they feel hungrier, causing them to eat more, which causes weight gain. In exchange for eating right, you become healthier and can enjoy weight loss."

Like the Zone, South Beach offers three, normal-size meals and two snacks each day. There is no need to count calories, weigh food portions or deprive yourself of tasty food. The diet works in three phases. The first two are restricted periods, and the third is offered as an ongoing lifestyle. Phase one is very similar to Atkins, restricting all carbohydrates, with dietary emphasis on lean meats, low sugar veggies, low fat cheese, nuts and eggs in order to maximize the rate of weight loss. In phase two, some of the banned foods are slowly re-introduced, while weight loss should continue. Phase three is a maintenance diet in which, having achieved your desired body shape, weight is neither gained nor lost.

On the downside, many of the medical statements made in Agatston's book, *The South Beach Diet*, have been challenged by other dietary authorities. For example, his alluring invitation to "lose belly fat first"—obviously something every dieting woman would love—seems implausible given the fact that the areas where we lose and gain weight on our bodies are largely determined by our genetic dispositions. Moreover, Agatston's diet is offered as a repeat formula. Whenever you gain weight, just jump back from phase three to phase one and start again. It sounds easy, but temporary weight loss offers no benefit and, as some experts argue, repeated dieting can be more damaging to the body than not losing weight at all.

Another controversy in South Beach doctrine is Agatston's statement that beer can't be allowed at any stage of his diet because it has a high glycemic rating and is loaded with maltose, a sugar derived from malted barley. Not so, says Anheuser-Busch, who took out full-page ads refuting the claim. Maltose is present in the early brewing stages of beer, but disappears during the fermentation process. As for the glycemic index of beer, one of the leading researchers in the field, Jennie Brand-Miller, author of *The Glucose Revolution*, has stated that beer has too few carbohydrates to assess its glycemic index, giving it essentially an index of zero.

Agatston has since changed his stance on the subject, saying that beer in moderation is acceptable in the later phases of the diet. South Beach, like Atkins and the Zone, is now very big business. Agatston's book has sold more than 8 million copies, and his diet is followed by celebrities like Bill Clinton, Nicole Kidman and Bette Midler. In a multimillion dollar deal, Kraft, the largest U.S. food company, is now tying more than 200 of its products to the diet. The maker of Oreos, Kool-Aid and Cheez Whiz will now have the South Beach seal of approval on brand foods lower in carbs and fats. The goal? Naturally, to lure shoppers back to Kraft's fold, since sales are flagging and many of its brands have suffered slumps as consumers slowly become more nutrition conscious.

• • • Blood Type Diet • • •

One of the keys to finding your own healing diet is to discover how much protein is right for your body, and one of the best ways to discover this is by using the Blood Type Diet as a guide. The best-selling book on the subject, *Eat Right for Your Type*, was written by Dr. Peter D'Adamo and published in 1996, but the work was pioneered by his father, Dr. James D'Adamo. It asserts that each major stage in our social evolution is associated with new environmental conditions and a different blood type.

Human beings began as hunter-gatherers, chasing herds of wild animals. Our main diet was meat and a combination of wild plants and roots, and we adapted genetically to maximize the nutrition from these sources. Our blood type was O, and D'Adamo maintains that people today who carry this type function best on a meat-centered diet. Wheat and dairy products were not developed at the hunter-gatherer stage, and so O types find them difficult to metabolize.

When we stopped hunting and started farming the land about 15,000 years ago, our diet changed dramatically from meat to a plant-based diet centered on grains, vegetables and beans, plus milk from domesticated cows. The genes of these agrarian peoples gradually adapted to a new way of eating and produced blood type A. People who carry this type function best on a plant-based diet. Of all the blood types, they are the most suited to vegetarianism.

Nomadic people emerged later and consumed a diet that was a combination of farm-produced plants and animal foods. This created a third blood type, B, for people who needed to be flexible in their diet so they could absorb nutrition from both plant and animal foods. According to D'Adamo, B types are better able to consume dairy products than O and A types.

And then, 900 to 1,000 years ago, the AB blood type evolved out of modern culture. AB blood types tend to be highly sensitive, rare and mysterious. They are destined for modern life and have the combined benefits of types A and B. ABs can usually tolerate a mixed diet in moderation, and do well with calming physical activity.

My experience with this diet is that there is a great deal of truth in it. People with type O blood tend to be more physically oriented, as hunter-gatherers once were, and have greater demands for protein. Also, type O people often have difficult metabolizing and digesting wheat. People with type A blood are frequently attracted to vegetarianism. B types do a little better than others with dairy foods.

But just as with other dietary programs, this one takes its basic premise to the extreme. People with O blood do not require the large amounts of animal foods that D'Adamo recommends. Beyond a certain point, protein is injurious to everyone's health, regardless of blood type, and is one of the reasons why we suffer from such high rates of osteoporosis, digestive disorders, heart disease, and breast, colon and prostate cancers. Most Americans already eat six times the amount of protein their bodies actually need, so encouraging O types to eat more is ridiculous.

In addition, we have all evolved to become dependent on grains, O types included, though they typically do better on brown rice, millet, quinoa and amaranth than they do on wheat and barley (the two high-gluten grains). It can be a major challenge to follow this diet in a family situation because it's hard to cook for two or three different blood types at the same time. Lastly, the rigidity of the diet can just be too unforgiving when, for example, an A type feels like eating steak, or an O type wants to live off raw foods for a while.

• • • Sally Fallon Diet • • •

Sally Fallon, a guest lecturer at our institute and author of *Nourishing Traditions: The Cookbook That Challenges Politically Correct Nutrition and the Diet Dictocrats*, believes in following the dietary traditions of our ancestors. Sally Fallon was inspired by the work of Dr. Weston Price, a dentist who knew nutrition was the foundation of well-being and traveled the world researching indigenous people's diet, teeth and overall health. He found that the further away people were from civilization, the healthier they were. They had fewer cavities and some cultures had never experienced or heard of cancer or heart disease.

Using Dr. Price's findings, Fallon studied societies throughout human existence and concluded that raw dairy products are an important part of a healthy diet. There are few subjects that raise as much controversy in the nutrition world as the subject of milk. Fallon argues that for the past 9,000 years, humans have relied on milk for their animal protein and fat. The problem with dairy, she says, is not the milk, but the modern methods used to make dairy cows produce the milk, such as selective breeding and the introduction of genetically engineered hormones. Pasteurization, thought by most to be beneficial, actually destroys enzymes, kills naturally occurring organisms that protect against pathogens and makes the proteins in milk difficult to absorb.

In dealing with another controversial subject, Fallon asserts that it is impossible to obtain adequate protein on a vegetarian diet. She cites studies of primitive cultures who relied on animal meat and had healthy bones, and claims that when agriculture was introduced, along with the consumption of grains and beans, health problems such as bone loss and tuberculosis appeared. Protein is an essential part of diet, and according to Fallon, animal food is the only source of complete protein, with all 22 amino acids necessary for the human body to thrive. Vegetarianism is now politically correct and many people advocate this way of eating, but since our ancestors ate animal meat, our bodies are meant to follow such a diet. She acknowledges that abstaining from commercial meats is a good practice, and that avoiding meat for a certain period of time can be cleansing and healing. But she cautions that strict vegetarianism can be dangerous, causing mineral deficiencies and health problems.

Fallon stresses the importance of the natural fats in meat, eggs and dairy, and encourages people to avoid the no fat or low fat alternatives to these products. In addition to high quality animal meat, she recommends other quality fats, such as virgin olive oil, unrefined flax oil, coconut oil and palm oil. Carbohydrates made from organic whole grains and treated properly to remove phytic acid, which is discussed further in chapter 7, are included in her diet. Additional essentials are high quality water, meat stocks, vegetable broths, unrefined sea salt, raw vinegar, fresh herbs and naturally fermented soy sauce.

The great thing about Sally Fallon is that she disregards the current fads and politics around food, and instead looks to our heritage to see what food is really best for human consumption. In modern, wholefoods nutrition, it's difficult to find people, other than the U.S. government and dairy farmers, who say that dairy is good for us, and her point about high quality dairy is a good one. On the other hand, her diet, so rich in protein and fat, is not what most Americans need right now. Americans are lacking vegetables and fruits, and consume six times the amount of protein they need (as mentioned earlier). Her suggestions may prove beneficial for many, but will not work for everyone.

• • • Raw Food Diet • • •

More and more people today are moving towards a raw food diet. Raw food is defined as food that is not cooked or heated. The basic premise of raw food theory is that we are the only species who cook our food and when we do, we kill the enzymes in it, denaturing the food and then ourselves when we eat it.

In its raw state, food is made of living cells. Cooked or heated food is seen as dead and lifeless because cooking kills the natural live nutrients and enzymes. It also changes the food's molecular structure, making it toxic. According to this theory, cooked food stresses the body as the liver, heart and kidneys all have to work overtime to eliminate the toxins ingested with the food. This leads to disease.

It is insisted that these cooked foods are also addictive and extremely difficult to give up. But once people do and start eating raw foods, they will experience clarity of mind, body and spirit. Raw foodists believe raw plant food is the only food humans should eat.

Raw food is very cleansing, healing and refreshing to the body, and is especially good for people who have eaten a lot of meat and processed food. Eating raw food may improve digestion and increase vitality. It is an environmentally supportive and ecologically friendly way of eating that can lead to a feeling of deep spiritual connection to nature. Going on a raw food diet can be like fasting for some, as it helps remove toxins quickly and effectively from the body and can lead to weight loss. One of the biggest benefits of going on a raw food diet is that it gets people off sugary, processed junk foods, which are all cooked.

This diet can be too cleansing for those whose systems are weak and need building. For people who have a sensitive digestive track, the intensity of the nutrients in raw food can be too much, and the cell walls of the vegetables may be too thick to break down and assimilate. The cooling effect of raw foods on the body makes this diet difficult to sustain during the winter months. People who are, to use a macrobiotic term, very yin—tall, thin, spacey—may need a more grounding diet as raw foods are very yin as well. It can be challenging to get adequate protein while on a raw foods diet. And too much sugar from raw fruits can lead to sweet cravings.

Some raw foodists are very adamant in their belief that cooked food is unfit for human consumption. Some are 100% raw, some 75% raw and some are 15% raw. Different people need different types of food, so I encourage people to experiment with the percentage of raw food in their diet, especially in the summer months.

• • • Master Cleanser • • •

The most popular cleanse out there today is the Master Cleanser or Lemonade Diet. It is a liquid monodiet, consisting of fresh lime or lemon juice, maple syrup and cayenne pepper with water. The drink is taken six to 12 times a day, and no other food is consumed during the cleanse. Stanley Burroughs, the creator of Master Cleanser, recommends it be followed for a minimum of 10 days, and up to 40 days, depending on a person's physical health. A laxative herbal tea, taken twice a day, and saltwater bathing are also recommended. Directions for coming off the diet include a slow re-incorporation of raw fruit, fruit juice, nuts and vegetables. Burroughs suggests doing the cleanse four times a year for optimum health.

The goal of the cleanse is to correct all health disorders. This lemonade drink was first shown to help aid stomach ulcers, and then Burroughs began to use it to help with other conditions. He says that as we eliminate or cure one disease, we correct them all and create vibrant health.

Improper diet causes the accumulation of waste, toxins and poison in the colon. These filter into the bloodstream and circulate throughout the body, inhabiting tissues and cells. The settling of these toxins weakens the cells and the entire immune system, opening the body to disease. Cleansing the body of this built-up waste rejuvenates its innate healing mechanisms. It then functions at optimal capacity, reducing toxicity, restoring health and vitality, and increasing our life force.

The Master Cleanser is an ideal way to cleanse and restore health because lemons and limes are a rich source of minerals and vitamins, are powerful cleansers and are available year-round. The unprocessed sugars in maple syrup provide energy, along with minerals and vitamins. The cayenne breaks up mucus and helps stimulate the digestive, respiratory and circulatory systems. Because the act of digesting food consumes our energy on an ongoing basis, the elimination of solid food for these short periods of time frees up this energy to aid detoxification.

Doing this cleanse—being free from coffee, tea, sugar, processed food and all food—is a freeing experience. Many people report that the cleanse was beneficial in helping them lose weight and feel healthier. However, a lot of people experience weakness, dizziness, nausea or even vomiting. According to the creators, this is the result of the poisons in the body being released.

It is common for people to decide they are going to fast in the springtime, especially if they've put on weight during the winter months. It's a pattern I have seen many times. They overeat during the holiday season and then, when the weather gets warmer and the days get lighter, they announce to themselves and everyone they know, "Okay, now I am going to clean it all up by going on a fast."

Being healthy is a daily practice. I do not believe that long-term fasting is an effective weight loss method. If you want to lose weight, just follow the simple instructions in this book and you are going to do so in a healthy, gradual way. Sudden fasts are a bit like going to pray once a week, instead of integrating spirituality into your everyday lifestyle. The way I see it, I fast half my life. Pretty much every day, I fast from 8:30 pm to 8:30 am. And I break my fast with my morning meal, called breakfast. This process has improved my digestion and my sleeping, and allows me to wake up in the morning with a greater appetite for food and for life.

There is no point in going on an extreme fast if you are unable to practice this simple form of daily fasting. Long-term fasting is a delicate and sophisticated art practiced by people who have already developed a certain ascetic habit of not eating as a spiritual discipline, beginning with short periods of time, then gradually extending to longer periods. It can be helpful for someone who is very ill with cancer, for example, to do a long-term fast, but for an ordinary person to jump to a 10-day fast will create a pinball effect, and do far more damage than good. Your body will think there is a famine and switch to survival mode, sucking up every calorie from the small amount of nutrients you give it. It has no idea that you have consciously decided to follow some program. And when you do break your fast, your body will put on weight more rapidly than before.

If you really want to fast, the best way is to cut out a specific, selected food, rather than reducing the quantity of food you eat. Just taking out one food from your diet can be a major undertaking. For example, you can decide to not eat sugar for a week. This is a very big deal. Just try it and see. Or, if you know you eat too much chocolate, just cut out this one item, and create a fast this way. You can also fast by adding food such as freshly cooked vegetables every day. As discussed in chapter 2, this can have the effect of crowding out other unhealthy foods. If you have success with this method of adding and subtracting things on your menu, you can begin to cut out more undesirable foods, one by one, or add more healthy foods, one by one.

When it comes to fasting and cleansing, remember that heroic activities may appeal to your mind, but can wreak havoc on your body. I suggest taking a middle path, doing things in moderation and realizing that your body doesn't necessarily know what your mind is thinking.

• • • Joshua's 90-10 Diet • • •

One of the things I began to notice in myself and others was that when we tried to eat totally clean and totally pure, we could only do it for a limited period of time. Sometimes it was a day, a week, a month or even a year. But at a certain point no matter how strong our idealism or willpower, certain foods we were avoiding became increasingly appealing. Once I started dreaming about those foods, it occurred to me that maybe my body was wanting something other than what my mind was permitting it to have.

At the time the Zone Diet was being introduced as the 40-30-30 diet, other nutrition experts were speaking about 40-40-20 diets and 50-25-25 diets. I began to think about how to express my new dietary theory in terms of percentages. Through that process, I came upon the 90-10 diet.

Since I'm not very much into rules, this dietary theory has only one rule. And even that rule is flexible. The rule is that 90% of the time you eat what is healthy for you, and 10% of the time you eat whatever you feel like eating. A lot of people try to stay 100% on their chosen diet program, which is bound to cause stress and likely to result in failure. There is no point in turning dietary "mistakes" into sins. Having fear and guilt around food is not healthy. Cravings are an opportunity to listen to the body and fine-tune eating habits. Instead of creeping guiltily to the fridge at 2:00 am for a pint of ice cream, publicly enjoy an ice cream with friends at an enjoyable social occasion, or get a delicious ice cream cone and eat it outside on a nice day.

• • • Finding the Right Diet for You • • •

All of these diet programs, and many more, are covered in greater depths in the school's curriculum. Students tend to get enthusiastic when we discuss the pros, then disappointed and confused when we reveal the cons.

"Which dietary theory is right for me?" is a question I frequently hear. But it's not about choosing the right theory. It's about finding what works best for you, then creating your own nutrition theory based on your individual desires and needs.

In chapter 7, I will explain the Integrative Nutrition Plan and you are welcome to explore that, too. But I don't want to give the impression that I am presenting all of these diet programs just to dismiss them and recommend my own. I want you to find the right one for yourself. This is a far more challenging task than getting swept away by the latest media-hyped fad and jumping on an already-rolling bandwagon. In the end, however, it will be far more rewarding because you will have come to understand yourself, experienced your own nutritional needs, and arrived at a place of lasting health and physical well-being. It is a very empowering experience for individuals to realize they don't need to follow someone else's guidance, but can control their own destiny, trusting their own intuition and intelligence. The result is worth the extra effort.

exercise

Create Your Own Diet

This is an invitation to create your own diet, based on what you have read about the previous programs and on other programs that you know. It will help clarify your understanding of how diets work, and what might work best for you.

1. List three major diet programs that appeal to you:

a. _Joshua's 90-10 diet_

b. _Ayurveda_

c. _~~Blood Type Diet~~ ~~macrobiotics~~ Raw Foods_

2. Write down five aspects of these diets that seem the most essential to you:

a. I like _Joshua's 90-10_ because _It's practical_

b. I like _Ayurveda_ because _I want to live in harmony w/ nature_

c. I like _~~Blood Type~~ ~~The Macrobiotics diet~~ ~~Raw Foods~~_ because _It includes (primary foods) lifestyle over all_

d. I like _Joshua's 90-10_ because _It avoids fear + guilt around food_

e. I like _Ayurveda_ because _It seeks balance_

3. Use these five qualities to create your own diet. Give your diet a name:

The _Best Self_ Diet.

Be creative! Try finding a name that will catch the public's imagination.

4. Make up your own rules.

The five most important points of The _Best Self_ Diet are:

a. _Identifying which types of food work well w/ your body_

b. _Making time for physical activity that you ENJOY_

c. _Significantly reducing or eliminating (crap) processed foods_

d. _Choose foods with low environmental impact_

e. _Be kind to yourself and others_

5. How long should your diet be followed? _A lifetime_

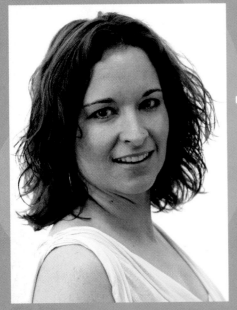

for eight years I worked as a management consultant
For eight years I worked as a management consultant
for Fortune 500 firms, always knowing I was meant to
do something bigger and better. After a lot of soul-search-
ing, I made the decision to finally follow my passion for the
study of nutrition and health. When my husband found the
magazine for Integrative Nutrition and brought it home, I knew
I had to enroll because its curriculum was so practical and
addressed the real-life questions people have about food.

Every weekend, I flew from DC to New York City to at-
tend class, and each time I never knew what to expect! In the beginning I thought I was going there
to learn about dietary theory, but I soon found out that Integrative Nutrition is so much more. I would
show up, get a bag of goodies (books, CDs, handouts and materials), and listen to Joshua and the
guest speakers. It was fun and educational at the same time, but what I learned the most about was
myself. I returned home from each class having grown into a little bit of a better human being.

The school told us to go out and get clients right away, and so that's what I did. As I worked with
my first few clients, my confidence began to grow until I became certain that what I am offering is
fantastic. I finished the school year with 14 clients and covered the cost of tuition many times over.

Since graduating from Integrative Nutrition, I have expanded my practice. I now offer one-on-one
coaching to 15-20 individual clients, as well as group nutrition "boot camp" programs. I also write a
monthly newsletter that includes articles, tips, recipes, and inspiration. I offer cooking classes and
corporate workshops. I am especially proud of the work I have done
with employees of the Embassy of Australia and the USDA. At the
Embassy I teamed up with another health counselor to offer a series
of ten wellness workshops that gave employees a solid foundation
to begin making healthy changes in their lives. The USDA has invited
me two years in a row to speak at their Food Safety Inspector Diversity Conference to speak on health
and wellness. For each of these engagements I was paid more than I ever thought I'd be paid for
doing something that is so fun!

Julia Kalish
Sterling, VA
Graduate 2004
www.innervoicenutrition.com

Going to Integrative Nutrition made me understand my body better and get in touch with what
I really want in life. For the first time, I understand the difference between doing what I really want to do
versus what I "should" do. The education at Integrative Nutrition made me see that I can have the life
I always dreamed about. Building on the confidence I gained throughout the year, I left my consulting
job a week before graduation and am now a full-time holistic health counselor. I love having my own
business. This work allows me to be open and trusting of myself, and gives me lots of free time. A
year ago I would never have thought this possible, but here I am enjoying the creativity and flexibility
of this amazing work.

chapter 4

Life itself is a yearning.
We yearn for meaning,
purpose, love, and
the fulfillment of our dreams.
Behind every human act,
no matter how singular or small,
is a yearning for more,
more life, more depth of experience.

The body also yearns.
It yearns for food, water,
touch, sound and sensuality.
It yearns for aliveness
through sweet things, tasty things,
and whatever stimulates and excites the senses
to a heightened experience of life.

Marc David

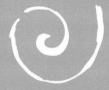

deconstructing cravings

CHOCOLATE, BREAD, STEAK, EGGS, French fries, candy bars, ice cream—it really doesn't matter what you crave. The important thing is to understand why you crave what you crave. Most people believe cravings are a problem, but I have a different perspective. Once it is determined that the body is a reliable bio-computer that never makes mistakes, programmed to be efficient and correct all the time, it is much easier to conclude that cravings are critical pieces of information that tell you what your body needs.

• • • Sugar-Addicted Client • • •

Many years ago, a successful female dentist came to me for help with her sugar cravings. She confessed that all day long she told clients to avoid sugar, but every afternoon she would sneak into her back office and secretly binge on sweets. She was a sincere, intelligent woman who knew that consuming large amounts of sugar destroys teeth, but was helpless when it came to her cravings. She was puzzled and felt helpless, not for a lack of understanding or discipline, but because willpower is not enough when it comes to food dependencies, especially sugar.

"I'm addicted and I feel like an absolute hypocrite," she told me.

"You're not a hypocrite" I said. "Humans naturally crave sweet flavor, but there is something you can do about it. Let's get some milder sweet foods into your diet on a more regular basis to avoid these afternoon binges."

I explained the distinction between simple and complex carbohydrates, advising her to reduce processed foods—except pasta, which she loved—and increase grains and vegetables. I knew, however, this alone would not be enough to beat her intense sugar cravings. So I introduced her to two new products, rice cakes and rice syrup. Rice syrup is a sweet syrup made from rice. It is processed, but contains an abundance of complex as well as simple sugars. Therefore, its impact on the body is much milder than standard candy bars, donuts and other processed, sugary foods. Rice syrup is delicious on rice cakes, which are puffed brown rice. They too are processed, but are also rich in complex carbohydrates. I told her to buy a big supply of rice cakes and rice syrup and put them in her back office for when she was craving something sweet. In two months, her sugar craving had diminished remarkably. She found the rice cakes and rice syrup adequate and satisfying. Months later, she was urging her own clients with sugar addictions to switch to rice products as a substitute for processed, chemicalized sweets.

• • • Simple and Complex Carbohydrates • • •

In today's nutrition world, high protein diets are fashionable and carbohydrate has become a dirty word, associated in many people's minds with the cause of obesity. This is absurd. Carbohydrates provide much of the energy needed for normal body functions—such as heartbeat, breathing and digestion—and for exercise. Carbohydrates are in everything from sugar to candy bars to grains and even vegetables. The problem is that people are not eating the types of carbohydrates nature intended. They're eating carbohydrate-rich foods that have been deformed, denatured and devalued.

All carbohydrates are made up of sugars. When sugar is digested it enters the bloodstream and becomes glucose. Glucose is fuel for all of the body's cells. Carbohydrates are considered simple or complex based upon their chemical structure. How fast the sugars enter the bloodstream and are converted into glucose depends on the type of carbohydrate. Complex carbohydrates are digested slowly. Simple carbohydrates are digested quickly.

Carbohydrates that appear in nature, as part of whole foods like vegetables and whole grains, are complex. Complex carbohydrates are composed of long chains of sugars. These long chains are bound up within the food's fiber. The sugars inside must be broken free from their chains and fiber to be released into the bloodstream. This is a relatively slow and methodical process. The sugars are absorbed into the bloodstream at a steady rate over the course of many hours, which is why complex carbohydrates provide long-lasting energy.

A very different process occurs with simple carbohydrates, which are in most modern processed foods. Other natural foods, like fruit, contain naturally occurring simple sugars, but because fruit is high in fiber, this helps slow down the digestion and limits the amount of sugar that floods into the cells. Processing carbohydrates strips them of all the bran, fiber and nutrients. Processed foods contain small molecules of sugar, unlike the long chains of sugar in complex carbohydrates, which enter the bloodstream momentarily after they are ingested. This causes a rapid rise in the glucose levels in the body—a sugar rush. The rush is shortly followed by a crash. The body sees the high level of sugar as an emergency state and works hard to burn it up as quickly as possible. Then blood sugar drops.

If you eat a whole grain—a complex carbohydrate—for breakfast, you will likely have energy throughout the morning, and then experience a dip around noon, just in time for lunch. If you eat an Oreo cookie, a candy bar or white bread, the bloodstream is suddenly flooded with sugars. You get a sugar rush as your blood sugar levels rapidly rise, but shortly afterward your blood sugar drops and you are hungry again. Your body naturally wants to maintain balanced blood sugar, so it is telling you to eat something to bring your blood sugar back up. Most people then go for more sugar and this process, of sugar ups and downs, goes on all day long. The most common time this happens is around 3:00 pm—a few hours after lunch. This is the time that most people crave sugar or caffeine to get through the rest of the day.

Simple sugars can lead to weight gain because our cells do not require large amounts of glucose at one time, and the extra sugar is often stored as fat. The anti-carb fad right now should really be an anti-simple-carb fad. If you want to lose weight fast, you don't have to go on a high protein diet. Just switch from simple to complex carbohydrates and eat lots of vegetables. You'll lose weight and improve your health. Plant foods are so low in calories that they force the body to burn its own fat. Nobody gets fat on a diet that's made up largely of green vegetables, sweet vegetables, whole grains and some low fat animal products. But throw in a bunch of cookies, white bread, French fries and a few quarter-pounders, and you've got yourself a weight problem.

• • • Kevin's Story • • •

A woman attending our school claimed to have a "problem child" named Kevin, who was significantly overweight and addicted to processed foods like sugary cereals, peanut butter and jelly on white bread, pizza, fast foods and all kinds of sodas and salty snacks. The more Kevin ate, the hungrier he got. This constantly ravenous 11-year-old was clearly eating too much, and overweight because of it.

I commented, "Maybe he's not hungry for calories. Maybe he's hungry for nutrition."

"What do you mean?" she asked. "I'm feeding him all day long. I would think he's getting too much nutrition."

I explained how the food he was eating is all processed, rich in simple sugars but deficient in nutrients. Sugar is fuel for cells, but they need vitamins and minerals to do their job properly. He was fueling his body, making his cells work, but not giving them the raw materials they needed. Kevin was craving more and more food because his cells were starving for vitamins and minerals.

I told her, "He's on a very inefficient diet and needs to eat a lot of food just to get enough nutrients to operate his body."

"What can I do?" the mother asked, now a bit stunned.

"He's got to reverse the formula," I said. "Eat foods that are rich in nutrients and low in calories, the exact opposite of what he's doing now."

I then laid out a program for her son, adding nutrient-rich foods like vegetables and whole grains to his diet, suggesting leaner choices of meat and plenty of exercise. Six months later, Kevin had lost 30 pounds.

Like a lot of people, Kevin was stuffing himself with sugary foods. Sugar cravings are as natural as our desire for air. During 2 million years of evolution, nature genetically programmed humans to desire sweet-tasting foods. Long before there was food processing, the only source of sweet taste was plant foods such as squash, tubers, roots, grains and fruit. In order to get the sweet taste the body desired, people had to eat plants. It is no coincidence these sweet foods are also great sources of nutrients, energy and fiber, everything we need to maintain health and survival.

• • • Foods Our Ancestors Ate • • •

Throughout history people ate food essentially as nature produced it. Food processing began relatively recently when people began harvesting honey and making whole grain flour, sugar, beer, wine and pickles. These foods were for special occasions, not everyday fare. People mostly ate whole and unprocessed vegetables, grains, beans, chicken, fish and other animal foods. It didn't matter if there were small amounts of sugar and honey or some wine and beer in the diet because there was physical work from sunrise to sunset for every member of the family. There were no cars, planes, trains or bicycles to get anywhere. Life was active.

It was only in the last century that massive food processing began. Gradually people found themselves eating more and more sugar. Sugar crept into everything from ketchup to toothpaste. Only 10 years ago you wouldn't find sugar in a natural food store, whereas today sugar is in everything, even in the health food stores. In addition, people started turning whole grain bread into white bread and brown rolls into white rolls. Pastries, muffins, bagels and donuts all came straight from the food processing plant.

The majority of foods in supermarkets are highly processed, including soft drinks, packaged snacks, already-prepared meals, boxed desserts and condiments. Nearly all these foods contain artificial sweeteners, colors, flavors and preservatives. Our ancestors would not recognize food in today's supermarket, especially those things eaten by children. A high percentage of children's diets are sugar, artificial ingredients and highly refined foods. The formative years of childhood are when good nutrition is most crucial, but our kids are eating junk, especially in the school system, and it shows. For the first time in human evolution, there is an obesity epidemic in children.

Most people don't realize the extreme effects of processed foods. Processing strips food of nutrients and even though some nutrients are re-introduced during fortification, there is no way a laboratory can re-introduce all the vitamins, minerals, carotenoids, phytochemicals and fiber that were originally in that food. A single tomato, for example, contains more than 10,000 phytochemicals. You simply cannot put all that back into a food after it has been taken out.

• • • Now, My Ice Cream Story • • •

I've been craving ice cream all my life, with a special sweet spot for Ben and Jerry's Cherry Garcia. One particular fall I noticed that on Sunday nights, after teaching class all weekend, my car would automatically swerve into the convenient store where I could buy a pint. As I watched myself eat all this ice cream, I wondered where this craving originated. "What am I doing in my life that might trigger such a craving?" I asked myself.

At the time, I was teaching a lot of hours and drinking hot tea to stay grounded and focused. I drank the tea without thinking, but pretty soon I noticed my body was feeling hot and tense. It wasn't long afterwards that I found myself craving ice cream. Teaching is, by itself, quite stressful when the hours are long, but I suspected that the hot tea might be adding to my condition. Also the hot tea, which I was drinking in much greater quantities than I was used to, might be causing me to crave cooling foods. I started drinking more spring water, and when eating in restaurants I stopped asking for water without ice. I also increased my intake of vegetables, which have a cooling and relaxing effect on the body, and olive oil to provide an alternative source of fatty satisfaction.

But I knew there were other contributing factors to my cravings. The fact that I would only have these cravings on Sunday revealed that I was using the ice cream as a reward after teaching all weekend. Also, my diet was mostly macrobiotic at the time, and I was eating very little fat. Both my parents consumed a lot of dairy growing up, and they were both around 75 years old and very healthy. I realized that dairy was a part of my ancestral diet and that my body was built to know how to handle dairy. With this knowledge, I increased my intake of organic yogurt products to get my fix without the added sugar and fat. And lo and behold, within a few weeks my cravings passed and I no longer needed my ice cream fix. I still look forward to eating it once in a while, but in reasonable quantities.

By observing my own behavior and trusting that my body needed something from the ice cream, I was able to modify my diet and lifestyle to get what I needed in a more health-supportive way.

• • • Cravings Are Not a Problem • • •

The lesson in all this is to look for the foods, deficits and behaviors in your life that are the underlying causes of your cravings. This may require a radical shift in perspective because many people view cravings as weaknesses, where in reality they are important messages meant to assist you in maintaining balance. It all comes down to trusting your body and its messages, rather than thinking of your cravings as the enemy, to be ignored and avoided.

How much do you trust your body? When I ask people this question, many reply, "Not very much."

"Why not?" I ask.

"Because it's always craving foods that get me into trouble," they say.

"What do you mean?" I ask.

"Well, whenever I'm on a diet my body wants foods that I'm not supposed to eat, foods that make me fat or sick."

"Why do you think your body craves such foods?" I ask.

"I don't know," people say. "I guess I've got some built-in flaws. I can't do the right thing when it comes to food."

The conclusion that the body is flawed when we cannot stick to some expert's diet is wrong. But it's a basic premise of almost every diet book. Without ever saying it explicitly, authors claim that if we want to lose weight and regain health we must control cravings for foods not on their diet plan. Success depends on conforming to the strict rules of this one diet. To do that we must develop deep discipline over our natural instincts. We accept this belief even though every other diet we have been on has been unsuccessful. We start the program with the best of intentions, determined to make good on this diet. Unfortunately, we soon learn that the part of us that directs our food choices cannot be disciplined, controlled, suppressed or denied.

We find ourselves increasingly craving illegal foods until one day we fall off the diet and feel guilty and worthless. We blame ourselves for failing to stick to the diet. It's not the program's fault, it's our fault. Or so we think. If only we could have been more disciplined, we would have lost weight and restored our health. It never dawns on us that there's nothing wrong with us, that maybe the diet theory is wrong.

This is how we come to believe our bodies or personalities are somehow flawed because we can't do what the experts told us to do.

Why is the instinct of human beings that determines food choices so powerful and unruly? Why can't it be easily controlled and disciplined? And what motivates these choices and cravings? Clearly, this is not a cerebral process. So what is it?

In my experience, the part of us that cannot be controlled is actually our inner guide to health and happiness. This innate wisdom is always trying to make us feel better by urging us to eat foods that will dissipate, if only temporarily, our physical tension, lack of energy and negative moods. In essence, this part of us is always monitoring our physical, emotional and psychological condition, and struggling to create balance, harmony and happiness therein. Cravings are the body's solution to such underlying imbalance, and food becomes a kind of medicine to regulate our current inner state.

Let me give a few examples. When we don't sleep well and wake up feeling lethargic, we often crave coffee to boost our energy and clear our minds. If we experience loneliness or mild depression, we often reach for chocolate or some other sweet food to boost our mood. After a stressful day many of us want to eat something sweet or drink an alcoholic beverage. After, we often feel weak and empty, and want something nutritious and strengthening. We crave eggs, steak, chicken or fish. These leave us feeling bloated and heavy. Thus begins a vicious cycle as we ping-pong from sweet, processed foods to excessive amounts of animal foods, from one extreme food group to another. Our minds, bodies and spirits are drained of energy, and there seems no apparent way out.

• • • Contracting and Expanding Foods • • •

I divide extreme foods into two categories:

1) Contracting

The most common and powerful contracting food is salt, which many of us consume regularly in large quantities. Salt is in everything, especially artificial junk food in brightly colored packages. Other extreme contracting foods are animal foods, including beef, pork, ham, hard cheese, eggs, chicken, fish and shellfish. The main benefit of animal foods is that they are rich in protein and provide us with feelings of strength, aggressiveness and increased physical and mental power. However, when we eat too much of these foods, we create an imbalance and quickly feel bloated, heavy, sluggish and slow-witted. The more contracting foods we eat, the more tight our bodies become. As a result of eating contracting foods, the body naturally craves expanding foods as a way of maintaining balance.

2) Expanding

The predominant extreme expanding food is refined white sugar. Expanding foods provide feelings of lightness, elevations in mood, relief from blockages and stagnation. However, refined white sugar causes rapid elevations in serotonin, followed by rapid declines. When serotonin levels fall, we typically experience feelings of depression, low energy, anxiety and loss of concentration. This is the moment when we crave extreme contracting foods to balance the equation. We then find ourselves in that ping-pong situation described above, bouncing back and forth between extreme foods, using one type to alleviate the effects of the other.

Our bodies can enjoy a certain quantity of extreme foods without necessarily creating too much imbalance. But when we exceed our personal limit—and it varies with each individual—there are consequences. If eating extreme foods is a daily occurrence for you, you are on the yo-yo diet, an exhausting process where you feel out of control as your body frantically tries to rebalance itself. To get out of this cycle, you need to deconstruct what you are craving, understand why you are craving those things, then find less extreme, healthier alternatives.

• • • Crazy Cravings • • •

Whenever your body is craving something, please pause and wonder, "What's really going on here?" Whenever you find yourself impulsively reaching for something you know is probably not good for you, take a moment to slow down, breathe and re-evaluate the situation. Consider what your body is really asking for. A good place to start is with flavor.

Are You Craving Something Sweet?

There are many forms of sweet foods, such as chocolate, cookies, pastries, sweet vegetables, fruit and fruit juice. As much as possible, try to satisfy your desire for sweet flavor with a milder, less extreme food than one that contains refined white sugar. Like my dentist client, try eating a rice cake with rice syrup on it. You'll be surprised how satisfying this treat is and how quickly it eliminates your need for extreme sugary foods. If something stronger is desired, try various cookies or pastries made from whole grain flour and sweetened with fruit juice or barley malt, a sweet syrup made from barley. The idea is to substitute a less extreme food that closely approximates the sugary foods you ordinarily turn to.

Certain vegetables have a deep, sweet flavor when cooked—like corn, carrots, onions, beets, winter squash (butternut, buttercup, delicata, hubbard or kabocha), sweet potatoes and yams. Then there are other, less popular vegetables that are semisweet—like turnips, parsnips and rutabagas. Eating a lot of sweet vegetables will satisfy your natural cravings for sweet foods, and reduce your cravings for sugary, processed junk food. A really simple way to cook these vegetables is by using a recipe I call Sweet Sensation, which you can find in chapter 7.

There are a few alternative sweeteners that are worth mentioning here. My favorite, and the favorite of most students at our school, is agave nectar. Agave nectar is a natural sweetener made from the juice of the agave cactus, the same plant that gives us tequila. But don't worry, there's no alcohol in it. The sweetness comes from a natural fructose that is absorbed slowly by the body. There is no sugar rush with agave nectar. It's great to have around the house to use in tea, salad dressings or when baking. Other popular alternatives to sugar are brown rice syrup, barley malt and stevia. All of these can be found in your local health food store and are talked about further in chapter 8. Try them and find the ones that work best for you.

Quality also makes a big difference. If you decide to have an extreme food, choose the best quality you can buy and there's a good chance you'll be satisfied with much less. Eat the food consciously, chewing it slowly and thoroughly enjoying it. Take chocolate as an example. Many of us crave chocolate and end up inhaling packages of M&M's or Hershey's kisses while on the run or at our desks. It is a much different experience to quietly indulge in a small piece of organic dark chocolate, thoroughly chewing each morsel.

Alternative Sweeteners

If you are a chocoholic, check out the chocolate section of your health food store and you will find many brands of organic chocolate, with many wonderful flavors. I'll talk about chocolate more in chapter 8.

Are You Craving Salty Foods?

Cravings for salty foods often indicate a craving for minerals. All salt originates in the sea, and natural sea salt contains 60 different trace minerals. Modern nutrition tells us that minerals are the basis for the formation of vitamins, enzymes and proteins. Common table salt, which most Americans use, has been refined and stripped of most of these minerals. People's diets are lacking in minerals because much of our food has been highly processed and chemically grown, hence the popularity of salty food. Before you go out and have a bag of pretzels or chips, eat a wide variety of vegetables, especially leafy green veggies, which are very high in minerals. This often satisfies the craving for salty foods that in fact is a desire for more nutrition. If your salt cravings continue, purchase a high quality sea salt to use in your cooking and incorporate sea vegetables, which have a naturally salty flavor and are high in minerals.

Are You Craving Bitter Foods?

Remember the saying, "It's the bitter pill that cures you"? Well, this is a good rule to live by, especially because the standard American diet does not contain many healthy bitter foods. Bitter foods enhance digestion, so when craving bitter flavor, your body is often craving nutritious foods that cut through fat and stagnation in the body's organs and digestive tract. Most people satisfy bitter cravings by drinking coffee and dark beers. If you find yourself craving bitter, try eating dark leafy greens, such as dandelion, mustard greens, arugula, kale and collards. These greens will unblock stagnant organs and promote healthy assimilation and elimination.

Are You Craving Pungent Flavor?

Chinese cooking often incorporates pungent-flavored foods that act as digestive aids. When craving pungent flavor, try grating fresh ginger on your vegetables or in your soup. In traditional Chinese medicine, ginger is an herb for the large intestine and lungs. It enhances function and promotes healing in both organs. Other foods with pungent flavor are cayenne, scallions, onions, leeks, garlic and pepper.

Are You Craving Spicy Foods?

Are you looking for an array of flavors, both subtle and strong, or are you looking for hot spices? So much of the American diet is lacking in flavor because it's been on the shelf a long time and is stale, bland and tasteless. These foods lack vitality, energy and aliveness. When fat and cholesterol are added to a diet of bland foods, the body becomes overweight and stagnant. Blood becomes thick, or viscous, and circulation slows. As circulation weakens, organs and extremities become cool. At this point, the body may start craving spices.

When people start wanting spicy foods they often turn to pizza or hot Mexican spices. These extreme foods warm the body, but also create so much chaotic energy that they stress the body. Instead of eating a pizza, with its dry, hard crust and heavy cheese, or refried beans and hot jalapeño peppers, try a bowl of noodles, such as soba, mixed with green vegetables and a nice marinara sauce that's got oregano, basil, onions, garlic and celery.

There are a variety of spices and condiments you can use to add kick to your food. Two popular choices are ground cayenne and hot pepper sesame oil, both of which you can find at any health food store.

What Texture or Consistency Are You Craving?

When craving something creamy, consider what you've been eating recently. Have you had a lot of bread, crackers or other baked flour products? When eaten in excess, these foods create feelings of dryness and stagnation. They also make us feel stuck, hard and irritable. When we reach that state of imbalance, we very often crave creamy, relaxing foods, such as ice cream, milk products or oily foods. Ask yourself if the texture that you're looking for is going to be satisfied by more oil, such as olive oil? Or are you looking for dairy foods like milk and yogurt? Try eating a salad with olive oil or some pan-fried noodles or vegetables with olive or sesame oil. To pan-fry, simply boil noodles and then put them into a frying pan with olive oil and sautéed vegetables. This simple recipe is delicious and very satisfying.

If you are craving chips or pretzels, it may be the crunch that you actually desire. The hormone that is released when we chew produces feelings of well-being, and the act of chewing enhances digestion. Instead of grabbing the chemicalized artificial potato products, try satisfying your crunchy cravings with raw carrots and celery, or organic versions of potato chips and hard pretzels with no added sugar.

Are You Craving Something Moist or a Liquid?

When craving liquids, ask yourself if you've been eating an excessive amount of salty foods or dry, baked flour products. Does your condition feel dry or tight? Are you thirsty? Many physical problems, including headaches, urology problems and kidney stones, are the result of chronic and habitual dehydration. People just don't drink enough water. Instead of quenching thirst with sugary and caffeinated beverages, try drinking high quality water at least three times a day. Put a bottle or a cup of pure spring water on your desk and sip it through the day. When the water enters your body, check in to how your body responds. If you suddenly awaken to how thirsty you are, then you know you've been ignoring your thirst. If you don't want the water, you will feel your body resist it, as if it were telling you that it has enough water inside and doesn't need anymore.

Are You Craving Something Crispy and Dry?

If you are craving something crisp and dry, maybe you've been drinking too many liquids. If this is the case, try to keep away from chips because they are rich in fats, especially saturated and trans fats, which cause heart disease and promote cancer. Avoid crackers that are highly processed and will elevate both glucose and insulin levels. To fulfill your craving for crisp and dry foods, choose rice cakes, high quality crackers without oil or sugar-free sesame sticks.

Are You Craving a Light or Heavy Food?

If you crave heavy foods, ask yourself if you've been eating a lot of salads or fruit. Are you cold, especially in the hands and feet? Salads, fruit and other raw foods make the body feel light. They also cool the body and can give rise to cravings for heavier, warming foods, such as fish, beef or hard cheese. Fish is rich in protein, low in fat and high in omega 3 fatty acids, which boost immunity and prevent heart disease. Likewise, if you are craving something light, go for some raw or steamed vegetables rather than a candy bar or other sugary snack.

Are You Craving a Nutritious Food?

So often when I find myself wanting to eat something, I check with my body to see what I am craving, and the feeling I get back is that I want something nutritious, something of substance. This is especially the case when I am working hard and utilizing the nutrition my body is getting from my diet. If you are hungry and nibbling on a raw carrot won't do, try a handful of trail mix, an avocado sandwich or one of those health food store bars made with fruit juice, nuts and whole grains. Later in the book there are some healthy snack recipes that you may want to try.

Are You Bored and Looking for Food to Entertain You?

We often use food to distract us from boredom. It's important to decipher true cravings from eating as a form of entertainment. If you are bored, try to deal with the issue directly rather than distracting yourself by snacking and munching to fill in time. Boredom is a challenge to be more creative with your life. I'll say more about this in chapter 6.

Are You in Need of Primary Food?

One of the biggest problems with diets today is that people attribute their cravings to appetite and hunger when they are really cries from another part of their being that is starving. These cravings have nothing to do with physical nutrition. These are cravings for what I call primary food, which is discussed in chapter 5.

Are You Needing Exercise Instead of Food?

Another common craving is for exercise. Stress, hard work and lots of thinking create tension in the body throughout the day. The body sends us signals that it's tense through body aches, tightness and constipation. Exercise is an ideal way of releasing that tension. All too often we attempt to medicate ourselves with food as a way of dampening unease and anesthetizing the body. Developing a regular exercise program to suit your particular body type and lifestyle will have numerous rewards. Start small. Go out for a walk, check out a gentle yoga or karate class. Listen to your body about what kind of movement it desires.

Are You Hypoglycemic?

In layman's words, hypoglycemia is the body's inability to handle the large amounts of sugar that the average American consumes. It's common among people with diabetes, but can also be caused by an overload of sugar, alcohol, caffeine, tobacco and stress. Hypoglycemia is triggered through the oversecretion of insulin by the pancreas in response to a rapid rise in blood sugar, which in turn causes blood sugar levels to plummet, starving the body's cells of needed fuel. A person with hypoglycemia may feel weak, drowsy, confused, dizzy and hungry, especially around 3:00 pm when blood sugar is naturally the lowest. When your blood sugar is low, you are vulnerable to cravings because your body urgently needs something to spike up its glucose. If a hypoglycemic episode hits you between meals, a healthy response is to nibble a carrot or celery stick, not grab a bagel with cream cheese or wolf down a chocolate chip cookie.

Physical health is the foundation of our lives. Once we free ourselves from extreme foods, the healing mechanisms of the body can concentrate on overcoming our deeper physical and emotional issues. That's when healing miracles occur. When people learn how to deconstruct their cravings, they can reclaim the sense of balance and bodily harmony that they were haphazardly seeking through indulgence or willpower.

What we crave, if recognized, acknowledged and accepted, will point us towards the food and lifestyle we need. In this way, our body is like a crying baby. The child is crying but it can't talk, so the mother has to figure out what has disturbed her child. Did it hurt itself, fall off a chair, not get enough sleep or wet its diaper? Is it teething or does it have allergies? The mother goes through a process of elimination until she finds the real problem. It's a similar situation with your body. Your body can't talk, but it can send you messages through discomfort or food cravings that need to be decoded.

For example, if you have a headache, try to figure out what caused it. Did you work too much in front of the computer yesterday? Did you not drink enough water? Did you drink too much wine at a party? Did you sleep with the window closed and deprive yourself of oxygen?

We can, and must, develop dialogue and relatedness with our body because it's talking to us all the time. And please remember, your body loves you. It does everything it can to keep you alive and functioning. You can feed it garbage, and it will take it and digest it for you. You can deprive it of sleep, but still it gets you up and running next morning. You can drink too much alcohol, and it will eliminate it from your system. It loves you unconditionally and does its best to allow you to live the life you came here for. The real issue in this relationship is not whether your body loves you, but whether you love your body. In any relationship, if one partner is loving, faithful and supportive, it's easy for the other to take that person for granted. That's what most of us do with our bodies. It is time for you to shift this, and working to understand your cravings is one of the best places to begin. Then you can build a mutually loving relationship with your own body.

exercises

1. Craving Inventory

For one week, keep a journal of every food you crave each day. Rate the craving on a scale of 1 to 10, with 10 being the strongest level of desire. Write down your thoughts next to each entry on how that craving is a response to an imbalance somewhere in your diet or life.

CRAVING	RATING (CIRCLE ONE)	TIME OF CRAVING	THOUGHTS ABOUT CRAVING
9/5 Sweet	1 2 3 4 5 6 ⑦ 8 9 10	9:00 pm	I've already had way too much sug ar today
	1 2 3 4 5 6 7 8 9 10		
	1 2 3 4 5 6 7 8 9 10		
	1 2 3 4 5 6 7 8 9 10		
	1 2 3 4 5 6 7 8 9 10		
	1 2 3 4 5 6 7 8 9 10		
	1 2 3 4 5 6 7 8 9 10		
	1 2 3 4 5 6 7 8 9 10		
	1 2 3 4 5 6 7 8 9 10		
	1 2 3 4 5 6 7 8 9 10		
	1 2 3 4 5 6 7 8 9 10		
	1 2 3 4 5 6 7 8 9 10		
	1 2 3 4 5 6 7 8 9 10		
	1 2 3 4 5 6 7 8 9 10		
	1 2 3 4 5 6 7 8 9 10		

2. Tongue Scraper

The tongue scraper, an inexpensive yet transformative utensil, is a simple, thin, u-shaped piece of stainless steel, with a well-defined yet safely blunted edge that removes gunk from the surface of the tongue. Dentists in America are recommending the tongue scraper more and more because it helps fight cavities by removing bacteria from the mouth. It also prevents against bad breath, especially for people who eat a lot of dairy and build up mucus in the mouth, nose and throat.

The tongue scraper comes from the tradition of Ayurveda, which asserts that people who use a scraper are better at public speaking, express themselves more thoughtfully, and speak more sincerely and authoritatively. Some people ask if the same effect can be gained by brushing the tongue with a stiff toothbrush. Brushing the tongue moves stuff around and is helpful, but a tongue scraper is more effective as it clears out the deep deposits and generally keeps the area more clean, stimulated and alive.

It also helps with cravings by cleaning the tongue of leftover food residue that could lead to cravings for those foods eaten previously. A tongue scraper reverses the process of desensitizing your taste buds, which has happened to everyone to a greater or lesser extent. It allows you to taste more subtle flavors in food so that you can eat vegetables, fruits and whole grains with greater joy. When old residue remains on the tongue, we aren't able to taste the natural flavors in whole foods. When you have a clean tongue, you will be better able to taste your food and won't need to eat as much since you will have gained greater satisfaction from your meal.

And finally, a big advantage is that it enhances kissing because it makes the tongue more sweet, fresh and sensitive. If you are in a relationship, I invite you to check this out with your partner. Make an agreement to scrape twice a day for one week, and feel the difference.

exercises continued >>

3. Dearest Body of Mine

Write a letter to your body, announcing your intention to listen more carefully to its messages and to act in a more loving way towards it. The following list of suggestions may be helpful to include, but be sure to make your letter personal to your own body. Set a specific period of time aside when you can sit quietly by yourself, undisturbed, in pleasant surroundings, and then begin to write. You don't need to complete the letter in one session. It is sometimes helpful to come back to your letter after a day or two, review the contents and make additions or subtractions. Write from your heart as well as from your mind.

Dearest body of mine,
After careful thought and consideration, I hereby promise to:

accept you and be grateful for you just the way you are
love and appreciate you for what you do
offer you healthy foods and drinks
overcome the addictions that hurt you
realize that laughter, play and rest help you feel good
exercise regularly and appropriately for my body type
adorn you with nice, comfortable clothes and shoes
understand that my unexpressed emotions and thoughts affect you
listen to the messages you are sending me when you are tired or sick
accept that I have the power to heal you
realize that you deserve to be healthy
honor you as the temple of my soul

_____

_____

_____

_____

_____

_____

I love you so much,

_____
please sign here

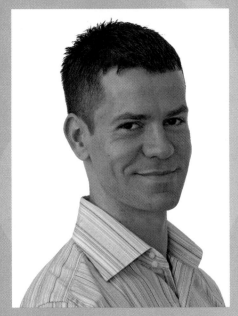

this time one year ago I had a day job as a business analyst in the computer field. I wasn't happy, felt very unfulfilled and had a deep desire to work in a career I actually enjoyed. Ultimately, I was searching for a way to integrate my ideas about nutrition, life and spirituality into a new profession.

Integrative Nutrition provided an excellent nutrition education and invaluable business advice. Step by step, I learned about the client acquisition process, how to work with clients, the places to successfully market my services and how to build a solid business foundation. Being in a community of supportive people who embraced me for who I am as an individual helped me feel confident that I could do this work.

Despite its reputation as a women's field, I found my niche in nutrition by specializing in gay men's health. I enjoy counseling men because they know I understand their particular concerns around sexuality and health. Being in school helped me realize the power in being a man, and I learned how to take charge of my masculinity while still embracing my sensitivity. This was a big breakthrough for me, and I am now able to help others through the same process. I'm truly empowering people in my community to have a better and more fulfilling life. And by seeing clients while still in school, I completely paid for my education before I graduated.

I am now a full-time health and life coach. I am the holistic health workshop facilitator for the The Institute for Gay Men's Health, associated with Gay Men's Health Crisis (GMHC) in New York, where I present several workshops each month. Many of the workshop attendees become my private clients. Also, I give health presentations at corporations, and have developed a three-month corporate group health program. Before coming to Integrative Nutrition, I practiced Reiki energy healing and taught pilates exercise. Now I've incorporated these specialties into my private practice. The combination of movement, food and energy work helps clients heal much more quickly than talk alone. My clients have all successfully learned how to have more energy, reduce stress, improve their self-esteem and eat a more nourishing diet.

Robert Notter
Graduate 2004
New York, NY
www.wholelifehealing.org

For the first time in my life I'm doing the work I am meant to do. The school reinforced that I have the power to create whatever I want with my life, and because of that I'm happier, healthier and wiser.

chapter 5

just as food is needed for the body

love is needed for the soul

osho

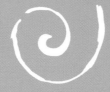

primary food

EVERYTHING IS FOOD. WE TAKE IN the experiences of life in thousands of ways that affect us physically, mentally, emotionally and spiritually. We hunger for play, fun, touch, romance, intimacy, love, achievement, success, art, music, self-expression, leadership, excitement, adventure and spirit. All of these are essential forms of nourishment. They determine the extent to which our lives feel enjoyable, fulfilling and worthwhile. In this chapter, I am going to talk about the differences between ordinary food and what I call primary food. Primary food is more that what is on your plate. Healthy relationships, regular physical activity, a desired career and a spiritual practice fill our soul and satisfy our hunger for living. If we are not physically starving, other dimensions of the human experience are much more important than what we put in our mouths, and this is why I refer to these dimensions as primary food.

When primary food is balanced and fulfilling, our lives feed us, making what we eat secondary. What is currently considered nutrition today is really just one source of nourishment, which I call secondary food. Secondary foods don't come close to giving us the joy, meaning and fulfillment primary food provides. When we use secondary food as a way to alleviate or suppress our hunger for primary food, the body and mind suffer. Weight gain is just one of the consequences. Disorders such as heart disease, cancer, obesity, high blood pressure and diabetes are national epidemics today, and one of the main reasons is because we are stuffing ourselves with secondary foods when we are really starving for primary food.

Think back to a time when you were passionately in love. Everything was exciting. Colors were vivid. Your lover's touch and feelings of exhilaration sustained you. You were floating on air, gazing into each other's eyes. You forgot about food and were high on life. Remember a time when you were deeply involved in an exciting project. You believed in what you were doing and felt confident and stimulated. Time was forgotten. Hours passed and you didn't even think about eating. Remember when, as a child, you were playing outside with friends in the evening. Suddenly, your mother announced dinner was ready, but you were not hungry. The excitement of play took all your attention. You were totally absorbed and not thinking about food.

Food doesn't cross your mind when you're in love, being creative or having fun. But when you're depressed, you may find yourself turning to food all the time for comfort and solace. Chronic depression is widespread in our society. So, too, are frustration, anger, disappointment, sadness and isolation. These conditions are all cries for primary food, but instead of giving ourselves these things, we often turn to secondary food. The problem is these substitutes don't work. If you are not getting the primary food you need, eating all the food in the world won't satisfy your hunger.

The importance of primary food became abundantly clear to me when I started a natural food store in Toronto. Sometimes after I closed the store at night, I would go to the movie theatre next door, where I noticed that many of the popcorn-munching, soda-gulping moviegoers looked happier and healthier than many of my customers. It became obvious to me that food was only half of the equation when it came to creating health. Eating well helps, but don't expect it to work miracles. It can fill you, but it cannot fulfill you.

Our institute divides primary foods into four main categories: relationships, career, physical activity and spirituality. I encourage you to look at these issues from a new perspective, as a form of nutrition.

• • • Relationships • • •

Over the course of a lifetime, we have many relationships—with parents, families, friends, teachers, lovers, coworkers and acquaintances. Just as there is no one diet that is right for everyone, there is no perfect way of relating that works for all people. What's important is to cultivate relationships that support your individual needs, wants and desires.

Friendships

I invite you to look at your relationships the same way people look at their wardrobes. You've probably kept many clothes you haven't worn for years. Maybe you are hoping they'll come back in style or maybe they are too small and, deep inside, you are hoping you'll be able to fit into them again some day.

It is the same with friends. If you write a list of everyone you know, chances are you will spot at least three or four people from your past who don't really belong in your present. In fact, if you're honest with yourself, you find their company draining. Maybe you've known them since high school, but now have nothing in common. Perhaps they are smokers and drinkers and you've moved on from that scene, past lovers who keep hanging around, needy people who want company and attention, or people who like to go out with you but when it comes to paying the bill forget to bring their wallets. My suggestion is to determine which of these people you can discard from your list. If breaking off all contact seems drastic, you can downgrade your relationship, see them less often and give them less of your energy. If this seems scary, don't worry. You're keeping your quality friendships and at the same time clearing space for new people to come into your life.

Now, using the same list, write down the names of three or four people you would like to spend more time with, people who are more of a contemporary mirror for you, who reflect where you are today, who have qualities with which you resonate. When you are clear who they are, be proactive and take initiative in increasing the level of contact. One of the easiest ways to do this is to invite each of them out for tea or lunch.

A key ingredient to the success of our school is community. Our students often make some of the best friends of their lives while in the school because they already have so much in common. They are healthy, happy people who want to do something that inspires them and helps others. Friends who listen and who are open can be difficult to come by. Having high quality friendships adds so much to life. If you want new friendships or to deepen current ones, I encourage you to write down the qualities you are looking for in a friend. Like any relationship, friendships take work, but can also be hugely rewarding. Remember, friendship is primary food. It should nourish you.

Love and Intimacy

We all need love. Love is soul food. Love is nourishment for the body, mind and spirit. To bring more love and intimacy into your life, I suggest deepening connections with everyone. Being close with others—husbands, wives, boyfriends, girlfriends, parents, children, friends, family and coworkers—is an essential part of life. Being free to express our hopes and dreams, fear and anger, joy and struggles with others gives us a sense of comfort, safety and connection that we do not have when we live in isolation.

When examining relationships, it is important to understand your personal preference in regard to how much intimacy you want or are comfortable with. It may be helpful to think about this on a scale of 1 to 10, with 1 symbolizing an individual who prefers very little social contact (a kind of monk-like state), and 10 symbolizing a person who enjoys spending a great deal of time with others. How do you rate on this scale? Avoid making judgments about which position is socially acceptable or superficially desirable, and take time to reflect where you are and where you really want to be. There are no rules, just personal preferences. We are all different.

There are people who love being alone, who feel energized by the experience, who require plenty of time to catch up with themselves. These people are relatively introverted and develop ways to be on their own with great ease. They usually prefer to relate with one or two people, and are finicky about who they choose to be their friends. At the other end of the spectrum are those who love having people around. These people are more extroverted, become energized by social interaction and often create an extended family and a network of friends. They look forward to seeing everybody at parties and holidays. Most people fall in between these extremes.

So, when I suggest improving the quality of your relationships, I am not saying everyone should be more social or get married. I am saying we need to find a type of love and intimacy that is appropriate and nourishing for us. It's a bit like establishing the ratio of carbohydrates, protein and fats that our physical body needs. Each of us needs to find a similar proportion of togetherness and aloneness in our social life, and know that this will change from time to time, just as diet does.

Touch, Hugs and Cuddles

It is known that a child who isn't held and touched enough won't grow to its full potential. Babies thrive on human touch, and holding them helps them become healthy, happy and well-adjusted. The same is true for adults. Most of us thrive on human touch, warmth and intimacy. Yet, most adults are touch-starved. We can get along in spite of this, but we may very well feel the lack.

It feels good to be touched, to be massaged, to feel connected. Due to a tendency to confuse touching with sexuality, many people today actually fear touch. In certain cultures it's common for women to walk arm in arm and for men to hold hands, but in Western society this is much less acceptable. Two men holding hands may invite the assumption they are homosexual. If women show too much love for each other, people will wonder if they are lesbians. Even if the sexual element is somehow removed, there is a layer of embarrassment or awkwardness around physical contact. It's helpful when people break through this social barrier and find comfortable ways to connect through touch. Think of it in the same way as a supplement: Be sure to get your recommended daily allowance of intimacy and touch.

It's not as difficult as you may think to find people who understand this need, who are aware that modern life is becoming increasingly isolating, and who want to connect and say hello in a warm way. Human touch helps us realize we're all in this crazy, modern world together. If you feel safe enough, you can massage someone's neck and shoulders as an exchange. You can do this with your partner, parents, children, friends and maybe even someone at work.

Sensuality and Sexuality

There are many degrees of physical intimacy, including touch, hugs, cuddling, sensuality and sexuality. It is important people understand what they're looking for in these delicate areas. It's not a small part of life, but somehow the whole issue of sensuality and sexuality, of love and relationship, just doesn't get discussed in an open, intelligent manner.

In a way, it's similar to our modern approach to shopping for food. Many people have no idea what's good for them, so they just pick brightly colored packages off the supermarket shelves. Similarly, people are confused about what they're looking for in relationship, and this increases the likelihood for misunderstanding, exploitation and frustration. Someone comes by, gives them attention, a warm hug, one thing leads to another and they feel like they're at the beginning of a relationship. They get super excited, making plans for the future and telling all their friends. Next thing they know, they're sobbing into a half-eaten pint of ice cream.

Sexuality and sensuality are an exciting and stimulating part of the human experience, and can be deeply nourishing and fulfilling if people get clear about what they want and how to communicate effectively to sustain the relationship.

Sex and Lovemaking

None of us would be here without sex. Sex created me. Sex created you. So, it's completely natural and normal that most of us are fascinated by sex. It doesn't mean there is anything wrong with us. If we weren't meant to enjoy sex, we would just touch index fingers or lay eggs to make babies. Or, at the very least, we would not be so full of hormones that from adolescence onwards we feel continually pushed towards sexual contact. Indeed, within the deepest and most evolutionary part of our brain, we are programmed to seek pleasure. Strangely enough though, the idea of sex as a source of primary food, as a nourishing, pleasurable and recreational experience, unrelated to childbirth, is relatively new, especially to women. Having a baby is a choice now that women have rights, economic independence and birth control. Sex is not just for making babies. Sex can be fun. Sex doesn't even require a significant other.

Masturbation has always existed, but was usually done in secret and cloaked in guilt. Recently, the idea of self-pleasuring has expanded and includes full permission for a woman or man to spend quality time alone, finding ways to create sensual and sexual pleasure in his or her own body. It can be a way to slow down and create a sacred and meditative environment, with candles, incense, gentle music and soft lighting. The freedom we now experience, living in a relatively liberal, democratic society in the 21st century, has given men and women the opportunity to nourish themselves with a wide range of sensuality and sexuality, two of the richest sources of primary food.

It may seem strange to be talking about sex in a book on nutrition, but we can eat an awful lot of broccoli and not get anywhere near the healing effects that come through great sex. What's needed is clear understanding and communication about what we want. A hug? A massage? A cuddle? A date? A relationship? A life partner? A child? If we want sex, how do we enjoy it? And it's no good waiting until we are already moving into lovemaking before deciding what we want because our mental machinery doesn't work very well once erotic feelings are aroused.

I invite you to use this section to ponder over what you want in terms of sensual and sexual nourishment, and to be creative, intelligent and adventurous in the ways that you get it.

Optimize Communication

A helpful exercise for couples is to talk about the positive and negative elements of their relationship. The best approach is scheduling a specific time when both are free of other occupations, with enough time and space to discuss delicate issues in a calm and sincere way. Begin with looking at the positive. Take turns. Each partner should speak, uninterrupted, for as long as he or she wants while the other listens carefully. Brag about all the aspects of your relationship that are going well, and allow yourselves to fully verbalize and appreciate each other. After all, you have found someone you feel close to, who you can relax and share your heart with. That is definitely something worth acknowledging and celebrating.

When you have both spoken, take a short break. Sit silently for a few moments, absorbing what has been communicated. Then, when you are ready, repeat the same structure, looking at one or two aspects of the relationship that you would like to see improved. It is important to communicate without blame, to express the areas of the relationship that aren't working or how you would like the relationship to grow. Maybe it's something simple, like household responsibilities, or maybe it's something deeper and sensitive, like wanting more quality time for intimacy and togetherness.

Problems can be more easily remedied when each partner clearly understands what the other wants. Sometimes, however, it proves difficult because one partner may want what the other cannot give. When this happens, don't fall into the trap of resignation. Instead, include the possibility of asking for outside help. We are not islands. We all have the same basic issues, and we don't have to deal with them in isolation. Counseling and support groups are available for every aspect of personal relationships. Remember, as you do this exercise, the aim is to strengthen the flow of nourishing energy that passes between two people. You are each other's primary food, and you are fine-tuning the recipe for long-term satisfaction.

• • • Career • • •

In today's society, most of us spend eight to 10 hours a day at work and very little time with our loved ones. But while we are choosy about who we relate with intimately, we spend years doing work we can't stand and may even be completely opposite to our personal values. Think about it for a moment. There are 24 hours in a day. We sleep for eight hours, work for eight to 10 hours and have six to eight hours left for other activities. Over half of our waking hours are spent working. Even more if we include commuting. It's a huge part of our daily routine, yet how many of us enjoy our work and how many complain about what we do, but feel powerless to change it? This not a nourishing lifestyle. No matter what food we are eating, if we dislike our job, it drains us of our health and vitality.

Somehow we don't realize the extent to which our lives would improve if we were doing work we loved. We have little to no understanding of our capacity to walk away from a particular job or career and begin a new one. In the flexible, fast-moving job market of today's business-oriented society, we can easily have three, four or five careers in a lifetime. Our parents and grandparents didn't usually have such choices. They knew one craft, one skill, and that was all they did. They were dedicated to the company, and the company was dedicated to them. We have the luxury of creating work that nourishes us and makes us want to get out of bed every day. I encourage you to take advantage of this, as it is essential to living a healthy, balanced life.

Finding the work you love

There is an exercise well-known in the field of job re-education called "Finding the work you love, loving the work you find." The first part, "Finding the work you love," goes like this. Make an inventory of all the things you love to do, including your hobbies, things that fascinate you, activities you enjoy in your leisure hours, and subjects you read about with great curiosity. Take your time; make sure the list is exhaustive. Somewhere in this list lies the key to your new career. Use it as an indicator of the kind of work you find enjoyable. It may involve food, massage, exercise, counseling or fashion. It may be hard to see at first, but in your hands you have the key to a new, exciting, creative career. When you have identified and selected your strongest interests, brainstorm on how you can blend these together to create a career that you love.

Loving the work you find

The second half of the equation is "loving the work you find." This relates to the job you are now in, and the potential for improving it as a source of pleasure and nourishment.

You may like your work, but carry resentment or disappointment because you are not paid adequately. How about giving notice? It could be your ticket to a new career or an increase in salary. Many students enroll at our school because they want to work in holistic health instead of their current job. They start seeing clients, enjoy the process, graduate, develop momentum to break through to a new career and go to their boss to give notice. I can't tell you how frequently they walk out with a pay raise. Sometimes all that is missing in an existing career is a 20% pay increase. If you give notice, and if you are a responsible, intelligent, hardworking employee, there's a good chance you'll get it.

One student was working for a large brokerage firm for many years, and they were keeping her working hours just under the requirement for full-time employment because this allowed the company to avoid paying for her benefits and insurance. She was fed up with the way they were treating her, and after months of thinking it through, she decided to quit. She walked into the office and announced she was leaving in two weeks. They immediately gave her the extra hours, switched her to full-time staff and bumped up her pay, saying they'd been thinking of giving her new responsibilities and more money anyway. She decided to stay on. "I wished I'd done it two years earlier," she confided in me.

Remember, we are spiritual beings living in a material world. We came to this world to accomplish something, which is probably not working in the office of a large corporation. We need to nourish ourselves by finding work we love and being paid fairly for it.

Notice how much our culture emphasizes the importance of money and career. A good way to get distance from this attitude and other self-limiting attitudes about work is to take a break for a year to travel the world. Go to exotic countries, see how other people live, meet other travelers, people who have found unexpected ways to mix work and leisure. Or apply for an internship in a new field that fascinates you. My encouragement to young people is that they be adventurous and take risks before they have the financial burden of supporting a family. Right now, young people, you've got time. You can explore and experiment, you can strive to develop a career in an area that stimulates you, rather than going for a safe but boring job.

There are few things more rewarding than being deeply involved in exciting work. You feel confident and stimulated, time stops, the outside world fades away. You are totally absorbed and energized by it. Doesn't it make sense to work on something you are passionate about?

• • • Physical Activity • • •

People need to exercise. Bodies thrive on it, and quickly degenerate without it. The challenge is to find the types of exercise you enjoy most, and then do them often. Physical activity can take simple and modest forms, like getting off the subway or bus one stop earlier and walking to your destination. It can be taking the stairs, instead of the elevator, to your office or apartment. It can be taking your dog for a walk or your children to the park. A 30-minute brisk walk every day may be all you need to keep yourself in shape. It's good to find something you can do every day without altering your schedule too much. Making physical activity a simple, daily habit greatly inceases your chances of staying active.

Something interesting I've noticed is people's inclination to choose exercise that aggravates their current condition. In gyms, the bulky, aggressive people tend to lift weights, which makes them more bulky and aggressive. Yoga classes are usually full of thin, vegetarian-type people who would probably benefit from doing some weight lifting, just as the weight lifters would benefit from doing some yoga. I am a big proponent of creating balance, and exercise is a great way to do just that. Different forms of exercise will give you different energy, and by listening to your body, you can find the kind of exercise that is best for you.

Please take a moment to consider your options. There are many. You can go rock climbing, paragliding, surfing, in-line skating or canoeing, or you can take up pilates, yoga, kung fu or kickboxing. You can find team sports like baseball or volleyball in which your daily dose of exercise is coupled with human interaction.

Spiritual nutrition is incredibly healing and powerful. Whether or not we feel we have a meaningful life plays an important role in wellness. Having a sense of belonging, a spiritual practice or something that gives us an underlying reason to be makes all the difference in our health.

I encourage people to have a spiritual practice, but in no way do I tell people what their practice should be. Some people follow their traditional religion of birth. Others explore Eastern religion or new age spirituality, or evolve an integrative approach. Personally, I say to myself that whatever makes the day turn into night and night turn into day, and winter become summer and summer become winter, and whatever keeps all the stars and planets going around perfectly in their orbits, creates new buds in spring and moves old leaves to drop away in autumn, can surely look after this one little life of mine. Seeing and experiencing myself as a microscopic part of the cosmos is what spiritual nutrition means to me. And by staying in harmony with the order of the universe, I tend to increasingly be in the right place at the right time, doing the right thing, just like all the other major elements in the universe.

Carl Jung popularized the term "synchronicity," indicating the presence of a subtle interaction between individual will and universal law, whereby a person can read the signs, see the way the wind is blowing, feel the direction in which life wants to go, and then use his or her creativity and intelligence to help it happen in the best possible manner. We always meet the right people at the right time to lead us to the next station in life. It can be incredibly rewarding once we develop a knack for noticing and welcoming synchronicity.

It's easy to embrace synchronicity when things are going well, but there are times when things seem to conspire against us. Some days the computer system decides to crash at the very moment I am about to complete an important document, and then there is a huge traffic jam when I'm in a hurry to get some-where. Three or four things all seem to conspire synchronistically, preventing me from doing whatever I think I need to do. At such frustrating moments all kinds of interpretations can pop into my mind, including the self-defeating attitude that life is against me. Life is never against me, or anyone. In these situations, the most effective strategy is to pause for a few minutes and reflect on the balance between the apparent antagonism of life in disrupting our plans, and the desirability and urgency of the goals we want to achieve. Maybe, on reflection, it's to our advantage that the goals are delayed a little, or maybe we're trying to push events faster than they can go out of an underlying fear that otherwise things won't turn out the way we want. Take a break. Step back. Reflect.

It doesn't mean that we have to abruptly give up all effort and swing to the opposite extreme, deliber-ately selecting signs and signals from these events to justify procrastination, or abandon our goals in favor of a temporary distraction like going to a party. Life is a delicate balance between two extremes, between will and let-go, between goal-orientation and spontaneous impulse, and we need to learn how to walk a middle path, be open to change, be sensitive to the natural flow of events, while not throwing away our own determined idea of where we want to go.

There are some good tools available to help develop such skills, including the Chinese masterpiece *The I Ching, or Book of Changes*, astrology, numerology, and dozens of tarot card decks. They can all help to bring you in tune, but don't take these tools too seriously; otherwise you may wind up relying on them to make simple, ordinary decisions. If you want to explore the same phenomenon without such tools, try creating a record of all the moments in your life when you felt synchronicity was happening to you: the people you met at pivotal moments by coincidence, the chances you took on a gut feeling, the decisions that somehow happened by themselves. When you have finished, see if you can apply this understanding to your daily life now, paying more attention to little synchronous happenings, like when the phone rings and it's the right person at the right time. You'll soon get the hang of it.

I encourage you to explore simple awareness exercises, such as watching your breath. While sitting in a relaxed, comfortable position, breathe through your nose and notice how the air is slightly cooler going in and slightly warmer going out. Place one hand over your heart and one hand over your belly. Feel your heart beating and thank your heart for all that it does for you. Feel your belly, noticing the rise on the inhale and fall on the exhale. Thank your belly for digesting all the food you eat. Sit silently, with your eyes closed, and allow yourself to be with yourself. Like yoga, it quiets the busy mind, relaxes the body, and brings a sense of being in tune with existence.

I could go on, listing other forms of spiritual practice, but in the end it all comes down to one thing: The more we take steps to bring our individual lives into alignment with the whole of existence, the more we feel nourished.

• • • Our Food Pyramid • • •

The Integrative Nutrition Food Pyramid illustrates the powerful synergy of primary and secondary foods. A symbol of our unique nutrition philosophy, it emphasizes the importance of high quality vegetables, fruits, complex carbohydrates, proteins and healthy fats. At the same time, the pyramid is surrounded with what is really vital in creating health—relationships, career, physical activity and spirituality. Secondary food, the food we eat, plays a critical role in our health and happiness, and discovering the food that is right for us is of utmost importance. But it's the four forms of primary food that truly nourish us and make life extraordinary.

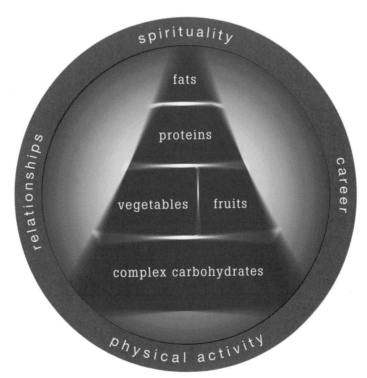

exercise

The Circle of Life

This exercise will help you discover which primary foods you are missing most. The Circle of Life has 10 sections. Look at each section and place a dot on the line to designate how satisfied you are with this area of your life. A dot placed at the center of the circle, close to the middle, indicates dissatisfaction, while a dot placed on the periphery indicates ultimate happiness. When you have placed dots on each of the lines, connect the dots to see your circle of life. Now you have a clear visual of any imbalances in primary food, and a starting point for determining where you may wish to spend more time and energy to create balance.

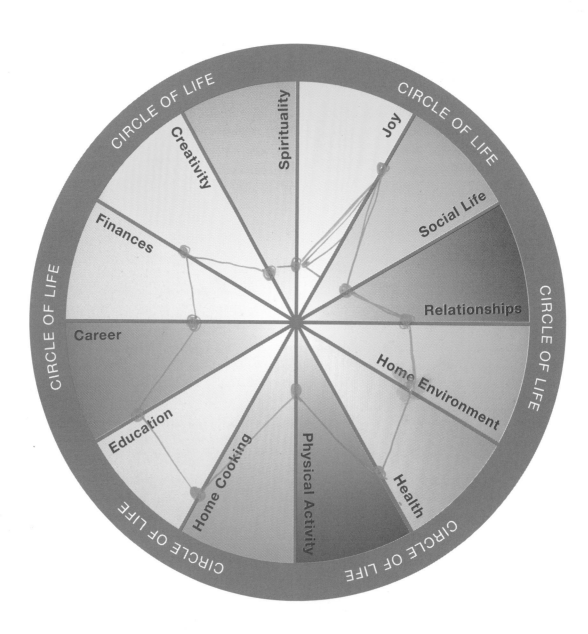

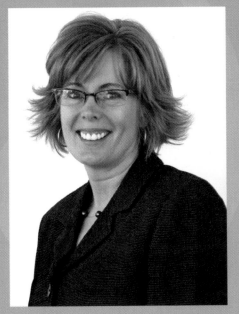

prior to enrolling at Integrative Nutrition, I maintained a 20-year career as a hairdresser and loved every minute. It was an incredible job with good hours, clients and monetary compensation. My life in general was also good: I had a strong spiritual practice, was eating well, exercising regularly, in a wonderful relationship and had two amazing adult daughters who were living and thriving on their own. One day I looked around my salon and realized there were no old hairdressers and I wasn't getting any younger. What was I going to do with the rest of my life? I knew it would take time to find an occupation I loved as much as hairdressing, and it would probably require some kind of training or continued education. As soon as I began my search, I stumbled across someone who had attended the school.

There are so many aspects of Integrative Nutrition that were life-altering. The most obvious and astonishing was overcoming my fear of public speaking. I was paralyzed by the thought of speaking in front of the class, which consisted of 60 people. Now I teach lectures in front of 300 people. This transformation would not have been possible without the support and patience of my entire class, the staff and Joshua.

Since graduating four years ago, my business has developed so much. I work with individual clients, long-distance clients all over the world, groups and corporations, and I hired two additional health counselors to help me with my growing client base. We currently have 60 active clients. I have developed a lecture circuit that includes one to three speaking engagements a week during the holiday season, and two or three times a month during the summer, if I am not on vacation. I have a core belief that making money should not interfere with down time. I am on track to earn $100,000 this year while working nine months at the most.

Rose Payne
Graduate 2001
Marlton, NJ
highlevelwellness@earthlink.net

I love this work. Each day is totally different than the day before. It never gets boring! Every day of my life is amazing. I'm about to be a grandmother for the third time. I just spent two weeks in Mexico with my life partner Chris, my close friend Gary (a guy I sat next to the very first day of class at Integrative Nutrition), and his partner. This summer, I'm going to India for six weeks. I have achieved my goal of finding a second career that I love even more than the first. I see myself doing this work forever.

chapter 6

Most people now begin realizing
that they live in the matrix.
What most people don't realize
is that the matrix lives in them.

Whenever we permit sodas, candy bars,
junk food, and cigarettes to enter our body,
we're letting the energies and vibes
of corporations, factories, offices, CEOs,
and executives into our very being.
These are the active ingredients of the matrix.

Zemach Zohar
www.alokhealth.com

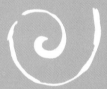

escape the matrix

What is the matrix? It's the old beliefs and false concepts about the world that drain our life force. The matrix is familiar and even comfortable, yet the beliefs and practices it demands of us steal our happiness and authenticity. The matrix repeats to us its rules about food, health and nutrition. We may live out a large portion of life never questioning what we've been taught, unaware of the beautiful reality that awaits us.

Escaping the matrix and reclaiming our own individuality and lifestyle is the task at hand. It is extremely challenging and rewarding. And, when you start to wake up and look around, you will find many other intelligent people on the same path.

So what does the matrix look like? Well, it's a kind of mental programming, driven by the corporate desire for profit that creates our collective beliefs about food, fashion and most aspects of life. The matrix looks like slender women who are young forever, virile men who are wealthy and powerful. It looks like an endless parade of things to buy, to play with, to wear and to consume. The matrix feeds on fast food, mass-produced junk, caffeine, sugar, white flour, meat, alcohol and medications that temporarily help us forget the pain we've created. The matrix has us running on stress, survival chemistry, and always tells us that we're not enough and that we need more. The matrix says we don't look good. It tells us not to trust others. It insists that we are really alone in this world. And it hypnotizes us to forget our true essence and greatness.

We may show our independence by making cynical, sophisticated remarks about aspects of the culture that surrounds us, about TV commercials or certain products, but in the end it is extremely easy to succumb to the overwhelming forces that bombard us every day with these messages. We willingly allow the clothing companies to brand us, eagerly abandoning our uniqueness as individuals and covering ourselves with logo-studded sneakers, pants, shirts, purses and jackets. Then we parade ourselves in front of each other, trying to gauge who has been branded best.

I have no desire to replace the free market economy or the democratic system with some revolutionary utopian ideal or any kind of socialist state. But it is ironic that in the years when Soviet and Chinese communism were viewed a threat to this country, our intellectuals went to great lengths to point out how brainwashing techniques and forms of social programming were being used in those parts of the world to control the behavior of millions of people. Yet people rarely pause to think what's happening here. In a slightly different way, this is also a form of "social-ism." It is an extremely powerful collection of attitudes, beliefs and thoughts that are being relentlessly imposed on the public, every day, in a thousand different ways. And the business-oriented motives that drive it are escalating out of control, causing damage to the mental and physical health of millions of people.

There are no real bad guys in this situation. Corporate heads are not evil monsters, cynically plotting how to exploit a gullible public. But corporations rapidly develop their own self-interested economic laws and dynamics because their survival depends on it. A fundamental economic law is that the corporation must always do what is best for the corporation. What is good for the corporation is to maximize profits, outperform competitors, expand, grow and keep shareholders happy with high-performance stocks and regular dividend payouts. Compared to these compelling dynamics, the health and welfare of the consumer is irrelevant. What's important is that the consumer buys the product.

Escaping the cultural matrix of needing to look, dress and eat a certain way means acquiring the courage to step away from outside influences, to look inside and ask yourself, "Who am I, and what do I really want from my life?" This addresses one of the most fundamental concepts embedded in the American psyche, the idea of freedom. We like to think we are the freest people in the world, and, in a way, we are.

As I see it, there are two types of freedom: freedom from and freedom for. Where "freedom from" is concerned, we are doing well. Through our democratic institutions, particularly the U.S. Constitution and Bill of Rights, we have achieved a great deal of freedom from religious persecution, from monarchy, from undemocratic political systems like communism, fascism and military dictatorships. But what is this "freedom for"? "Freedom for" what? To work our butts off all day and then sit in front of a TV, computer or play station until it's time for bed? To stuff ourselves with processed food until our pants burst or our bodies deteriorate? To chase after the latest products that will make us feel complete? Isn't there something more to life than this?

• • • Hungry? Why Wait? • • •

One of the most insidious features of the matrix is that it tells us that life is about instant gratification. And if life is about getting what we want as fast as possible, then so is food. In fact, if the nutrition problem in America today had to be summed up in a single sentence, this one-liner from a commercial for Snickers bars might be the most succinct—"Hungry? Why wait?" Introduced to the market almost 80 years ago, Snickers is now the number-one selling candy bar in the U.S. due to savvy marketing techniques based on familiarity with people's snacking habits.

As the slogan implies, there's no need to wait until the next meal, no need to bother preparing and cooking food, or waiting for other family members to get home to sit down together for a meal. Just grab the nearest tasty thing and pop it in your mouth. Modern marketing and distribution have ensured that when we feel hungry, there are many available products lining the shelves of the local stores or stacked in the office vending machine. Almost all these foods are loaded with calories, trans fats, refined sugar, processed salt, dairy products and artificial chemicals—foods not fit for human consumption.

One Snickers bar has 280 calories. The ingredients listed on the wrapper are as follows: milk chocolate (sugar, cocoa butter, chocolate, lactose, skim milk, soy lecithin, artificial flavor), peanuts, corn syrup, sugar, skim milk, butter, milk fat, partially hydrogenated soybean oil, salt, egg whites and artificial flavor. I have nothing against Snickers bars. I even ate one a few years ago, but I'm using Snickers as an example of the way people are being seduced into buying foods that, when eaten regularly over time, increase weight and decrease health.

The job of advertising, a multibillion dollar industry, is to stimulate the buying impulse of the biggest consumer society on the face of the earth. We are constantly bombarded with ads encouraging us to eat and drink more. From the billboard on the side of the bus to the back cover of a stranger's magazine on the subway, from commercials slotted between songs on the radio to the ones that interrupt our favorite television shows, we are exposed to an overwhelming inundation of commercial messages every day.

Remember Joshua's Law of Advertising? The less healthy a food is, the more money will be spent on its marketing. There is an average of 200 junk food ads in four hours of children's TV during Saturday morning cartoons, the prime time for kids to be watching their favorite programs. The number of 30-second TV commercials seen in a year by an average child is 20,000, and the number-one ranking advertiser for child-oriented advertising on television is the junk food/fast food industry. No wonder childhood obesity rates are skyrocketing.

I'd like to make it clear that I am not against fast, convenient food. I think it's a great idea. But I long for the day when the colorful packages on our supermarket shelves and the papery wrappers from fast food restaurants contain good, wholesome, nutritious foods that keep us healthy. It is possible. All we need is for enough people to demand it. Then instantly, overnight, the companies whose existence depends on knowing what we want and supplying it will switch to healthy products in order to guarantee their own survival. It's really up to us.

I've said it before and it's important to remember that what we're dealing with here in the U.S. today is something totally new. Nothing like this massive consumer society of ours has ever happened in the history of humanity, and it's very possible that nothing like it will ever happen again. This message of mine may seem simplistic. Maybe you think you're aware enough to see beyond the Madison Avenue glitz and hype, but the ads keep coming, they keep entering your brain, their influence is powerful and seems to be escalating. Can you be vigilant enough in your own life to filter out the useless messages that the matrix communicates?

● ● ● The Pressure to Be Thin ● ● ●

The idea of being thin enters girls' minds very early in life. Most girls in the U.S. own a Barbie doll, and Barbie has a body shape that is impossible to attain. If women were really built like Barbie, they would not be able to walk, have a menstrual cycle, give birth or breathe. We may like to think our modern culture is beyond looking up to Barbie as a role model, but if our young girls see this doll as an image of what it is like to be a woman, what kind of message does that send to them about how they should look? Increasingly, young girls say they want to be thinner and claim to be dieting.

The world needs strong, powerful, nurturing women to stand up and counterbalance the overly masculine modern society. Most women are, by nature, nurturing. But so many women are bound and silenced by their insecurities because of the messages they have received throughout their lifetimes about what it means to be female.

Try reading a women's fashion magazine and you will see the content and advertising are incessantly inflaming, and cashing in on, obsessions with seeking to measure up to media-driven images. The pages are covered with emaciated women. And these are the people that our society agrees are beautiful. These models are idealized, and the advertisements make us want what they've got so that normal women will go and buy those Louis Vitton handbags or Ralph Lauren sunglasses to feel attractive.

What is shown in magazines, however, is not reality. There are no disclaimers announcing that the models work for hours with the world's best hair and makeup artists, that the clothes are tailored to fit their exact shape, or that the photos are retouched by professionals. Blemishes are removed, cellulite wiped out, any extra fat from the belly, thighs, arms or wherever is erased. Women see these ads and somewhere begin to believe they are supposed to roll out of bed being as beautiful as these models on the pages of the magazine.

Supermodels represent the cutting edge of all that is supposed to be beautiful and desirable in a woman. But they come from another planet. Most models are thinner and taller than 99.9% of all American women. The average model is 5'11" and weighs 117 pounds, whereas the average American woman is 5'4" and weighs 140 pounds. To keep their jobs, models must maintain zero body fat. Take a moment to digest these words: zero body fat. The human body, especially the female body, is simply not designed to operate with zero body fat. It's an inhuman concept. Small wonder that, on any given day, more than half the women in this country are on one diet or another, trying to mold themselves into an artificially created cultural concept of what it means to be beautiful.

Even now, in the 21st century, the female half of the population continues to experience oppression, in a very real way, on a daily basis. Women are being squeezed between two powerful cultural forces. One is the pressure to consume readily available, unnecessarily fattening foods, and the other is the pressure to conform to a female stereotype that demands slimness as a prerequisite for beauty. In both cases, advertising is the key to unlock their minds and purses. Marketing is the catalyst, the trigger that stimulates and provokes them to buy both the unhealthy food and the unhealthy American feminine beauty ideal.

Advertising encourages women to substitute food for love, while glamorizing images of borderline anorexic women. The media is reluctant to examine the impact of advertising on the public's health for the simple reason that it depends on advertising for commercial viability and cannot afford to bite the hand that feeds it. As we already discussed in chapter 1, government is compromised by the power of corporate America, so really there is no one left to protect the public, no one even to speculate that perhaps the public might be in need of protection. Left to ourselves, we can just drift along with the collective cultural mind-set and try to make the best of it, or we can choose to stand up for what we know is the truth regardless of what the media wants us to believe.

• • • Superwoman Syndrome • • •

Another pressure many women find themselves dealing with is the superwoman syndrome. Liberated from the confinement of traditional female roles, with increasing opportunities to explore areas that were once exclusively for men, women frequently end up leading chronically stressful lives as they struggle to balance all their options. They want to be successful in business, have a great marriage, beautiful children, a dynamite figure with a flat belly, involve themselves in the arts and maybe even run for office some day. Phew! Just thinking about it makes me stressed out. Many women who seek counseling with me and attend my school create this lifestyle for themselves, and then wonder why it's not making them happy.

I am a great believer in encouraging people to slow down. I understand why women want to explore all the possibilities open to them, having been denied them so long, and I admire those who manage to do so. But sooner or later anyone who maintains such a high-powered lifestyle, man or woman, is bound to see that an intelligent selection of priorities is required. Courage is also needed to stand up and say, "Okay, everyone. You can pass me on the fast track to success. I've tasted it, understood it, and I am no longer interested in keeping up because I know now that the price is too high. I want to stay true to myself, and I want to enjoy myself. These are my priorities."

• • • Superman Syndrome • • •

As the director of a school with 90% female students, I tend to focus on the sexual oppression of women more than men. But men today also have enormous pressure to be perfect, to be strong, to take care of the family and provide, and to be there for their women or lovers. In recent years, marketing geared towards men has dramatically expanded to include images of men with fit bodies, including six-pack abs, who are also successful in their careers.

When we teach sexual oppression at the school, I am always reminded of the pressure men feel around responsibility. Just as women are seen as "sex objects" in our society, men are seen as "success objects." Somehow, men in our culture get the message that if they don't "bring home the bacon," and in large quantities, they are failures. And if anything goes wrong, it is their fault. Many men carry guilt from things that happened years and years ago that, in reality, were not their responsibility. The drive to be a success object often causes men to override their bodies. They don't listen to the wisdom of their cells, to the gentle voice inside that would have them be more gentle, slow and self-loving. After all, by our culture's standards, this isn't very manly.

In helping men overcome the pressure to be perfect—to have a fit body, a well-paying job and to be open, but not too sensitive—I encourage men to find people with whom they feel relaxed. I urge them to create communities in which they feel comfortable to be themselves, without the pressure to conform to other people's ideals of who or what they should be. Lastly, I support them in letting go of any guilt or responsibility for things that may have happened in the past.

Men in our culture are ready to learn that they don't need to sacrifice their bodies. Males are often expected to lay it all on the line, to sacrifice their health to toxic jobs and to the army, to push themselves with pride and take injuries or wounds "like a man." Yes, men can be strong, but they can also be vulnerable. Many men want to nourish themselves, to be caring around their own health. They need encouragement and permission not only from the women around them, but from their fellow men.

• • • The Individual • • •

How does all this translate into day-to-day reality for a health educator like me?

Well, for one thing, my emphasis is personal, not general. Even though I have to look at the big picture, at the structure of the matrix surrounding us, my focus is always on the individual sitting in front of me, and on listening carefully with an open mind to what she or he is saying. This is something I picked up from Zen Buddhism. It's called "Zen Mind, Beginner's Mind," and refers to the art of approaching something with an innocent attitude, in a fresh, receptive and inquiring manner. This is a wonderful way to starve the matrix and let the beauty of the truth of who we really are shine through.

I look at the person who has just walked into the school as tabula rasa, a clean slate, trying not to impose any of my personal prejudices, and I ask, "How are you? What is your health concern?" There is a lot of evidence in counseling that, without the counselor making any recommendations, a person will get themselves well just by speaking about their problems and receiving love and attention. This approach takes time and runs counter to mainstream healthcare, in which the focus is to get the job done quickly by diagnosing symptoms, identifying diseases and prescribing medications.

Looking back, I notice that many of my clients recovered quickly, and I attribute this to my careful listening skills, my deep appreciation for them and my deeper knowing that they need not suffer. In fact, many of my clients and students could probably have worked out their problems themselves, without my help, providing they were willing to put as much attention and intelligence into their own healthcare as they do into their work. But somehow this rarely happens. Society, culture and media all shift people away from caring for their own health, as if it's boring or uninteresting compared to other aspects of their lives. Instead of investigating what's "inside here," they are trained to focus on what's "out there," such as fashion, the lives of celebrities and gossip.

Integrative Nutrition reminds people to love themselves, be with themselves and respect themselves. We teach people to notice the issues that are troubling them, and then invest time and energy into creating a healthy, happy life. Our method makes people focus on themselves and address the issues that are bothering them. Once this happens, the solution is usually quite obvious, and the person with the answers is usually the individual, not the professional. But having that person there, a trained listener who is devoted to helping them get better, is how people discover their answers.

• • • Fitting Out • • •

One of the more powerful ways we can free ourselves from the matrix is to learn to "fit out" rather than trying in vain to "fit in." We are all susceptible to this age-old social pressure to conform, to be accepted and do well in the eyes of others. This feeling of needing to fit in drives us at high speed towards a poor diet and fast foods, and straight into addictions to energy-boosters like coffee and sugar. Having become a slave to our own ambitions, we then feel compelled to push forward with all our life force. Getting off this treadmill requires a willingness to stand alone and disregard opinions of others.

I am personally sensitive to this tendency because, being Jewish, I grew up with an inbuilt ethnic survival instinct, a protective understanding that you don't want to get caught, you don't want to attract unnecessary attention, you need to pretend you're just like everyone else. That's why I easily spot the same tendency in others. I have noticed that people who have already shifted to significantly different lifestyles sometimes try to hide it or play it down for similar reasons.

A lot of the people who become students at our institute don't fit in normal society. In one way or another, they live on the periphery and don't want to attract too much attention, so they mimic the customs and habits of their families and neighbors. They readily tell me, "I am nothing like my brother or my sisters, my parents, or my next-door neighbors. I see myself as being quite different from the society around me." But they'll blend in with the crowd, chatting about the latest election, sporting event or social happening, and wear the same clothes, just to be acknowledged as part of the collective.

Marriage is an area where we often compromise for the sake of appearances. After three years of marriage, I knew mine wasn't working for either of us. But I stayed married for another three years because my parents were so happy that I had married a Jewish woman. I could not imagine disappointing them. This same pressure manifests in a thousand different ways, and our eating habits—at home, at the office or in the restaurant—are sure to reflect our willingness to compromise for the sake of social harmony.

I'd like you to pause for a moment and reflect on how much of your intelligence and creativity is being channeled into "fitting in." My own experience is that if you put the same amount of effort into "fitting out"—giving yourself permission to be spontaneous, natural and authentic in the way you live and behave—you'll immediately become much happier and more content.

Escaping the matrix is a key step in creating true health and happiness. Start by noticing the places in your life where you feel you are inauthentic. Are there certain people who you have difficulty expressing your true self around? In what circumstances do you try to fit into other people's expectations? Without self-judgment, begin to notice when and where this occurs, and start building the confidence to express your true self at all times, to embrace what makes you different from the norm. By loving yourself completely, you will reach a new height of health that no food could ever give you. And by expressing your authentic self, your life force will soar, your heart will open, and the world will never look the same.

exercises

1. Turn Off the Media

I encourage you to hide your TV for one week. Don't read magazines or newspapers, and avoid the Internet and listening to the radio. Notice how your thoughts about the world and about yourself change without constant media messages.

Write down all the media you are exposed to on an average day and all the messages you receive. Be sure to include radio commercials, television commercials, billboards, Internet ads, subway ads, etc.

Television shows _____

_____

_____

_____

_____

Magazines or newspapers _____

_____

_____

_____

_____

Advertisements _____

_____

_____

_____

_____

_____

_____

2. Wish List

This is a tool for you to get in touch with all your deepest desires—from relationships to feelings to vacations, anything at all.

Step One: Start listing your desires. Begin with simple and obvious desires, and you will notice that more ideas come to you once you start writing. Allow yourself to go crazy—write down all that you desire. Use any language you are comfortable with, such as "I want…" or "I desire…" or "I intend…" Allow yourself to run free.

Step Two: Whenever you fulfill a desire, put an "x" in the "Done!" column. In the "Gratitude" column, thank anyone who may have helped you attain your desire. You might be thanking yourself.

WISH	DONE	GRATITUDE
1 I want to do more yoga		
2 I want to go climbing more (inside or out)		
3 I hope to surround myself with a community of likeminded people		
4 to live authentically		
5 to create a fullfilling & economically thriving buisness		
6 to travel to different countries for work & pleasure		
7 I want to be a loving & present parent		
8 I hope to improve my self confidence		
9		
10		
11		
12		
13		
14		
15		
16		
17		
18		
19		
20		
21		
22		
23		
24		
25		

3. Hot Water Bottle

At bedtime, place an old-fashioned hot water bottle on your belly for about 15 to 20 minutes. The lower belly is the home of your Hara, the central balance point of your body, and according to Asian philosophy it is the center and source of your life energy. Hara is the gate, the doorway to the universal energy surrounding us. Heat from a water bottle brings more energy and more blood circulation to these digestive organs, which are really the engine of your bodily vehicle. It aids in digesting food and in unblocking energy that may be stuck after a heavy meal.

On a psychological and emotional level, warmth on the belly may promote absorption and digestion of whatever feelings or mental input are left over from the day's events. It's an ancient and natural feeling for both men and women to seek some kind of warm coziness at nighttime, and if there isn't someone in the bed then a hot water bottle can help create this feeling.

I get a lot of feedback from single people about how they dread getting into a cold, empty bed at the end of a busy day. After being introduced to the hot water bottle solution, some of them even start using two or three of them to create a soothing, comforting feeling that helps them relax and sleep better. It's a simple and effective way to feel nourished.

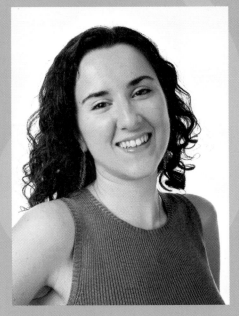

I was studying at John Hopkins with the intention of becoming a gynecologist when I was diagnosed with polycystic ovarian syndrome. I weighed two hundred pounds, had cystic acne, depression, and had not been menstruating for years. The medical community had nothing to help me, and at the same time I realized that I didn't want to work with women through the traditional medical model. Feeling lost about what I did want to do, I went into corporate America, where I had a variety of high-level marketing positions in start-up technology companies. When I discovered Integrative Nutrition, I was ready to get back to my passion for creating health.

It was great having exposure to out-of-the-box thinking around health and nutrition. The school was so cutting edge compared to my previous educational experiences, which were archaic and textbook-based. I was amazed by how all the authors I was reading in books and health magazines were coming in and talking to us. The community of students was out of this world, and the experience of opening up to them was life-altering.

I knew my body wanted to get well and that I could heal if I figured out how to give it what it needed. The only thing that worked was playing with my food. As a result of changing my diet, I lost 60 pounds, cleared my skin so that it glows, and have not missed a period for four years. I did all this without medication, supplements, herbs or vitamins—just food! My sense of well-being was restored, and that is priceless. But beyond self-empowerment, I was opened to the possibility of going out there and empowering others. The school encouraged me and gave me the tools to become a holistic health counselor, from a nutrition and business standpoint.

I have been working full time as a holistic health counselor for four years now, and it's been fantastic. I am the founder and director of Laughing Sage Wellness Group, where I have two other health counselors as my associates and our niche is helping women with

Alisa Vitti
New York, NY
Graduate 2002
www.laughingsagewellness.com

menstrual and sexual health issues, such as polycystic ovarian syndrome. One out of four women has PCOS, and it goes mostly undiagnosed by gynecologists. The medical community has nothing for these women, so it's great to be able to offer my assistance, creating synergy with their doctors. I do a lot of public speaking and I have been requested as an expert on women's holistic healthcare for television. I am thriving, and I don't even work as much as most people do.

Personally, this work continuously inspires me to live a balanced life. I have plenty of time to cook, get away on the weekends, and am always finding new ways to express myself authentically.

chapter 7

A journey of a thousand miles

must begin with a single step

Lao Tzu

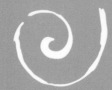

the integrative nutrition plan:
12 steps to health

WE'VE EXAMINED THE POLITICS surrounding the food industry and the difficulty of breaking out of contemporary cultural attitudes that influence our eating habits. We've looked at the innate wisdom of the body, learned to trust it and to understand the importance of signals it sends to us in the form of cravings. We've examined dietary theory and looked at the pivotal issue of primary food. Now it's time to integrate this knowledge in the form of a plan. No one way of eating will work for everyone, but this is a program of general principles and suggestions, not rigid rules. There is flexibility to include variations according to each individual's needs, recognizing that no two people are alike and no two people have the same food preferences.

I do not expect people to change their way of eating all at once. On the contrary, I have found that drastic, sudden shifts make it difficult to maintain a new diet because they force people to repress their food cravings and imbedded eating habits. The more these are repressed, the more powerful they become, producing internal stress that builds until people fall off the wagon and the diet fails. A gradual introduction allows people to implement changes without as much effort or strife.

Gradual Sustainable Change

Even by choosing just one step from this chapter, significant changes will occur for you. Think about it like climbing a ladder. It is important to take one rung at a time because if you take too many steps at once, you're more likely to fall off. I am making many suggestions, but it is up to you to find the ones that fit. Most diet books recommend that you completely alter your current way of eating and follow their strict rules. I say choose the things that you most want to do and leave the hardest one for last because as you start doing the easier ones, your body's energy will kick in and you will pick up momentum. You will then find yourself doing the hardest one with greater ease because you're not starting from zero.

If you like the hot towel scrub, do that. If you want to eat more sweet vegetables, do that. Whichever suggestion you want to follow is the right one for you. One thing I can tell is they all work.

There are 12 steps to the Integrative Nutrition Plan, but there is no special significance in this number and you do not need to follow the steps in order. Pick one step and then go to another when you are ready. Go at a pace that's suitable for you. You could tackle one new step a day, a week or a month. This isn't a short-term diet; this is a long-term lifestyle. Trust your instincts, and know that each change you make has a tremendous impact on your present and your future.

The 12 steps are as follows:

Drink more water

Practice cooking

Increase whole grains

Increase sweet vegetables

Increase leafy green vegetables

Experiment with protein

Eat less meat, dairy, sugar, chemicalized artificial junk foods. Less coffee, alcohol and tobacco.

Develop easy and reliable ways to nurture your body

Have healthy relationships that support you

Find physical activity you enjoy and do it regularly

Find work you love or a way to love the work you have

Develop a spiritual practice

Some of these steps are dealt with more extensively in other chapters, but I will summarize them here to give a sense of overall continuity and completeness.

• • • 1. Drink More Water • • •

The body is 75% water, so it makes sense that this essential fluid must be continually replenished. We can go for a month without food, but we can live only two or three days without water. This really illustrates how crucial water is to our survival.

Being told to drink more water may leave you wondering, What is "more"? What is the correct quantity of water for your body? Some experts say eight glasses a day is the right amount, but this leads to the question, How big is one glass? Eight ounces? More? Less? The true answer must come from your own experience. Much will depend on whether you are a big person or a small person. A smaller person will need proportionally less water than a bigger person. It also depends on your level of physical activity, the climate and your diet.

 Increasing water increases yin, making the body light and airy and expanding energy through the whole system. If you are too yang—too tight or contracted, suffering from stress, headaches and bodily tension—you may want to try increasing your water intake to balance these symptoms. In addition, cravings for sweet, yin foods may actually be signals of dehydration. Drinking water may reduce or eliminate the cravings.

I recommend either bottled water or filtered water. Most tap water contains chlorine, fluoride and sometimes even lead. If you drink bottled water, try all the different brands available and see which is best for you. Don't just settle for the cheapest one. Good water is like good wine; it requires careful selection, plus sensitivity to how your body responds. If after researching water filters you decide to invest in one, be sure to change the filter regularly, in accordance with the instructions.

Timing is also important to water intake. After waking up in the morning, it's good to drink one or two glasses of water immediately to hydrate the body. Many people, in the evening, realize they didn't get their eight glasses, so they drink a lot right before bed. Good sleep is integral to health, and is disturbed by waking up to go to the bathroom. Certain deep states of sleep, necessary for rest, relaxation and regeneration, occur only when we sleep deeply. You may not be able to comfortably hold much water in the bladder for long periods of time, so if you notice that you are waking up at night to go to the bathroom, I suggest drinking most of your water in the morning and early afternoon.

Many diet consultants say water is the only liquid that can hydrate the body, and that juice and tea don't count, but for me it's caffeinated drinks that don't count because they are dehydrating. Herbal tea, soup and juice all help hydrate the body, although not as much as pure water.

Some people say they can't drink water because they don't like the taste. My advice to them is do whatever it takes to make it taste good, like add some fruit juice, a squeeze of lemon, a slice of cucumber or anything that creates an appealing flavor.

Dietitians sometimes recommend drinking hot water with lemon first thing in the morning, claiming it's good for cleansing the liver. If you do this, don't take it as absolute truth, but see how your body reacts. There is no one recommendation that works for everybody. If you're already a stressed and tight kind of person, lemon may pucker you up and make you tighter. Experiment and see what really works for your body at this point in time.

The same thing applies to ice water and hot water. A lot of people refuse ice in their water because they think it's unhealthy. On the other hand, they may think nothing of drinking pints of hot tea, thereby creating an overheated condition, which the body, through its natural wisdom of seeking balance, will need to compensate for by eating something cooling, such as ice cream.

There are certain foods that are more water-dense than others. Cooked grains are two parts water, one part grain. Vegetables also have high water content. Steaming or boiling vegetables, as opposed to frying or baking them, further increases their water content. If you eat a dry breakfast cereal or bread, a muffin or cookies, you will take in little or no water from these foods. In fact, they may create a water deficiency, while cooked grains, vegetables and soups may create a surplus.

Considering the impact of water on human health, it amazes me that people remain so unaware and uneducated about this subject. They spend most of their lives dehydrated, needlessly suffering from low energy, cravings and symptoms, not realizing they could feel much better by merely drinking more water.

• • • 2. Practice Cooking • • •

In Zen communities, the role of chef is traditionally given to experienced, esteemed monks because they understand the wisdom of proper food preparation and the effect it has on the entire community. As I mentioned earlier, I was fortunate as a child in that my mother would take me food shopping with her, we would come home and unpack the groceries, and she would teach me how to cook certain foods. My mom was a relatively lazy cook and would whip meals together in just minutes. This was helpful for me to see because I learned that cooking could be relatively simple.

It takes virtually no time to cook, but this realization usually comes only after a lot of experimentation. It's a bit of a paradox that only a skilled cook knows how to prepare a meal in just a few minutes; you would think expertise would bring complexity. But making a meal can actually be divided into two, simple stages: preparation time and cooking time. Preparation time for rice is short, about a minute. Take it out of the bag, measure it, rinse it and put it in the pot. Cooking time is longer, but this doesn't mean you need to hang around the kitchen, impatiently testing the rice every few minutes to see if it's ready. Just flip on a timer and go about doing whatever else you need to do.

Vegetables, which are the ingredient most missing from the modern diet, are especially easy to prepare. Making a salad involves only rinsing and chopping. Cooking vegetables takes a couple of minutes of prep time—to rinse and chop—and then a few minutes of cooking time—to steam, sauté, boil or bake. Juicing is an instantaneous way to prepare vegetables; all you need is a juicer and a few minutes to clean it once you are done.

Learning the art of simple meal planning will help you get all the nutrients you need as well as release you from dependency on restaurant food, fast food, other people's food and processed food. We eat differently when we are feeding ourselves than when we are out and about. Restaurant food is usually very salty and highly flavored as it's designed to be a taste sensation. And it often comes in very big portions. By buying and preparing our own food, we eat more accurately according to our body's actual needs. We are less likely to overeat or consume as much salt and flavoring.

Being capable of preparing delicious, satisfying meals in a brief period of time is a skill worth learning. It's not difficult, but it takes practice. You may burn the rice or overcook the kale. You have to go through an initial period of trial and error. Give yourself permission to make mistakes. It's like starting a new office job. The first week or two seem complicated because you have to figure out how the phone system works, how the photocopy machine works, where the bathroom is and who's who in the office. In the beginning it seems like a huge task, but a month later you are doing it without even thinking about it. You know it all by heart. Cooking is just like that.

For many people, the task of cooking seems daunting. They are puzzled, and ask questions like, "How do plain, ordinary vegetables turn into such a delicious meal in a few minutes?" A chef is like an alchemist, turning simple ingredients into gold, transforming a caterpillar into a butterfly. But few cookbooks talk about the initial, challenging period. They don't mention that cooking a meal takes much longer when you are an inexperienced chef than after you have practiced.

It is a great gift to be able to cook with ease and confidence. In just a short time you will be effortlessly washing, chopping, cooking and nourishing yourself and others. And if there is one skill you want to be good at, it is to know how to feed yourself and those you love high quality, delicious food, because this will change everything. Cooking is an art because it involves creativity. When you creatively select certain combinations of foods, it's similar to a painter choosing colors from a palette. Cooking is one of the highest forms of art because it's the only art that actually enters the bloodstream and becomes who you are. You can look at a painting and find it inspirational, hear a piece of music that creates a certain mood, but with homemade food, there's a much deeper effect. Besides its beautiful outside, the food actually enters into your body. There's a very intimate relationship between a meal and the person who consumes it.

• • • 3. Increase Whole Grains • • •

Many fashionable diet theories today are advising people to avoid carbohydrates. These theories make carbohydrates the villain and the main cause of weight gain. But this is a huge generalization. Looking at the delicate, thin bodies of many Japanese people who are on high carbohydrate diets, composed of large amounts of rice and starchy vegetables, it's impossible to conclude that all carbs lead to weight gain.

Whole grains have been a central element of human diet since the beginning of civilization, when we stopped being hunter-gatherers and settled down in agrarian communities. People living in these communities, on all continents, had lean, strong bodies until very recently. In the Americas, corn was the staple grain that people ate. In India and Asia, it was rice. In Africa, people had sorghum. In the Middle East, they made pita bread, tabouli and couscous. In Europe, it was corn, millet, wheat, rice, pasta, dark breads and even beer that were considered health-providing foods. In Scotland, it was oats. In Russia, they had buckwheat or kasha. Very few people were overweight.

The reason people are gaining weight is because they eat too much chemicalized artificial junk food, and take in too much caffeine, sugar, nicotine and alcohol. They are taking in things that lead to weight gain or that cause cravings for foods that do. It's not simply the carbohydrates. If they were eating bowls of freshly cooked whole grains and vegetables every day instead of processed junk food, people would not be getting fat. Oddly enough, people today will eat all kinds of junk food, as long as it is low carb or no carb, but they refuse to eat whole grains, which might significantly benefit their health.

Whole grains are some of the best sources of nutritional support, containing high levels of dietary fiber and B vitamins. And, because the body absorbs them slowly, grains provide long-lasting energy.

Creating great grains

• Measure the grain. Rinse. Remove any unwanted material.

• Optional: Soak for 1 to 8 hours, which will eliminate phytic acid and make them more digestible. Drain the grains and discard the soaking water.

• Add grains to recommended amount of water and bring to a boil.

• A pinch of sea salt may be added to all grains except amaranth, kamut and spelt (it interferes with cooking time for these).

• Reduce heat, cover and simmer for the recommended time.

1 CUP GRAINS	WATER	COOKING TIME
amaranth	2½ cups	20 minutes
brown rice	2 cups	50 minutes
barley	2–3 cups	60–90 minutes
buckwheat (kasha)	2 cups	20 minutes
bulgur	2 cups	20 minutes
cornmeal (polenta)	3 cups	15 minutes
couscous	1 cup	5 minutes
kamut	3 cups	5 minutes
millet	2–3 cups	30 minutes
rolled oats	3 cups	30 minutes
whole oats	3 cups	1½ hours
quinoa	2 cups	20 minutes
spelt	3 cups	2 hours
wild rice	2 cups	1 hour

All liquid measures and times are approximate. It's a good idea to check your grains halfway through and towards the end of cooking to determine if they are done or more liquid is needed. If too much liquid has been added, remove the lid and boil off excess. You can change the texture of grains like quinoa, millet and buckwheat with different cooking methods. Bringing the liquid to boil before adding grain will keep the grains separate, like rice. Boiling grain and liquid together creates a softer, porridge-like consistency.

Cooked grains keep well, and some grains take a considerable time to cook. For this reason, busy people can cook extra grains for later in the week. To reheat cooked grains, simply add a bit more liquid and reheat gently on the stove.

As mentioned earlier, whole grains can help Americans with one of their basic health problems, an inability to maintain an even level of blood sugar. Whole grains release sugar into the bloodstream slowly, similar to an IV drip, as opposed to the sudden rush caused by consuming sugary foods and sodas, which in turn cause surges and crashes of energy.

Sally Fallon, whose diet was discussed in chapter 3, points out that people traditionally soaked or fermented their grains, often for a few days, before cooking. All grains contain phytic acid in the outer layer of the bran. Phytic acid combines with certain minerals in the body, such as calcium, magnesium, copper and iron, and can block absorption in the intestines, which may lead to digestive disorders, mineral deficiencies and bone loss. Soaking grains or fermenting them—by soaking in hot water with vinegar—neutralizes the phytic acid and makes the grains easier to digest. Eight hours of soaking in warm water will neutralize the phytic acid, and greatly improves the nutritional benefits of grains. Even an hour of soaking will help. If you have difficulty digesting grains, you may want to try soaking them overnight to see if it improves their digestibility.

The most common grain in our culture is wheat. Many people are allergic to wheat, but don't know it. Wheat products are heavily marketed by the government in the food pyramid and in the food industry with all the breakfast cereals, cookies, cakes and crackers. Gluten—a protein in wheat, barley, rye, buckwheat and oats—is difficult to digest. If you are sensitive or allergic to gluten, you will experience bloating, constipation and/or gas after eating wheat and other glutenous grains. Other related symptoms are allergies, celiac disease, brain fog, chronic indigestion and candida. Sometimes the symptoms occur immediately after eating, but they can take time to manifest. If you think you have sensitivity or allergies, I recommend removing all wheat and gluten products from your diet for four to six weeks. See how you feel.

● ● ● 4. Increase Sweet Vegetables ● ● ●

Almost everyone craves sweets. Rather than depending on processed sugar, adding more naturally sweet flavor to your daily diet dramatically reduces cravings for sweets. Certain vegetables have a deep, sweet flavor when cooked—like corn, carrots, onions, beets, winter squash (butternut, buttercup, delicata, hubbard and kabocha), sweet potatoes and yams. There are other, less popular vegetables that are semi-sweet—like turnips, parsnips and rutabagas. Then there are vegetables that don't taste sweet, but their effect on the body is similar to sweet vegetables. These include red radishes, daikon radish, green cabbage, red cabbage and burdock. They sooth the internal organs of the body and energize the mind. And because many of these vegetables are root vegetables, they are energetically grounding, helping to balance out the spaciness people often feel after eating other kinds of sweet food.

A simple way to cook these vegetables is to follow the recipe below that I call Sweet Sensation. It has few ingredients and preparation time is minimal.

Sweet Sensation

- Use one, two, three, four or five of the sweet vegetables mentioned above.
- Chop the hardest ones, like carrots and beets, into smaller pieces.
- Softer vegetables, like onions and cabbage, can be cut into larger chunks.
- Use a medium-sized pot and add enough water to barely cover the vegetables. You may want to check the water level while cooking and add more water if needed. Remember, vegetables on the bottom will get cooked more than the ones on the top. Cook until desired softness. The softer the vegetables get, the sweeter they become.
- You may also add any of the following ingredients: spices, salt, seaweed. You can add tofu or a can of beans for extra protein.
- When cooked to your satisfaction, empty the ingredients into a large bowl, flavor as desired and eat. The leftover cooking water makes a delicious, sweet sauce, and is a healing and soothing tonic to drink by itself.

Other delicious ways to incorporate sweet vegetables into your daily diet include eating carrots raw, baking sweet potato fries, roasting squash, making soup with corn and onions, or boiling beets to put on top of your salad.

• • • 5. Increase Leafy Green Vegetables • • •

If vegetables are the scarcest ingredient in the American diet, green vegetables are lacking most of all. When we nourish ourselves with greens, they naturally crowd out the foods that make us sick. Learning to cook and eat greens is essential to creating health. Greens help build our internal rain forest and strengthen blood and respiratory systems. They are especially good for city people who rarely see fields of green in the open countryside. Green is associated with spring, a time of renewal, refreshment and vital energy. In Asian medicine, green is related to the liver, emotional stability and creativity.

Nutritionally, greens are high in calcium, magnesium, iron, potassium, phosphorous, zinc, and vitamins A, C, E and K. They are crammed with fiber, folic acid, chlorophyll and many other micronutrients and phytochemicals.

Some of the benefits gained from eating dark leafy greens are:
- blood purification
- cancer prevention
- improved circulation
- immune strengthening
- subtle, light and flexible energy
- lifted spirit, elimation of depression
- promotion of healthy intestinal flora
- improved liver, gall bladder and kidney function
- clearing of congestion, especially in lungs, and reduction of mucus

There are so many greens to choose from. Be adventurous and try greens you've never heard of. Broccoli is very popular among adults and children. Each stem is like a tree trunk, giving you strong, grounded energy. Rotate between bok choy, nappa cabbage, kale, collards, watercress, mustard greens, broccoli rabe, dandelion and other leafy greens. Green cabbage can be included as a green, either as sauerkraut, which provides the body with live enzymes, or as an ingredient in the Sweet Sensation recipe. Then there are arugula, endive, chicory, lettuce, mesclun and wild greens. These are generally eaten raw or in any creative way you enjoy. Spinach, Swiss chard and beet greens are best eaten in moderation because they are high in oxalic acid, which depletes calcium from your bones and teeth, leading to osteoporosis. Cook these vegetables with something rich like tofu, seeds, nuts, beans, butter, animal products or oil. This will balance the effect of the oxalic acid.

Cooking Greens

Try a variety of preparation methods like steaming, boiling, sautéing in oil, water sautéing, pressed salad and waterless cooking. Boiling makes greens plump and relaxed. I recommend boiling for under a minute so that the nutrients in the greens do not get lost in the water. You can also drink the cooking water as a health-giving broth or a tea, if you're using organic greens. Steaming makes greens more fibrous and tight, which is great for people who are trying to lose weight. Raw salad is also a wonderful food. It's refreshing, cooling, soft and supplies live enzymes.

When most people hear "leafy green vegetables," they probably think of iceberg lettuce, but the ordinary, pale lettuce in restaurant salads doesn't have the power-packed goodness of other greens. Get into the habit of adding these leafy green vegetables to your diet as much as possible. Try it for a month and see how you feel.

• • • 6. Experiment with Protein • • •

Protein is good for us. It's the basic building block of the human structure, helping to form muscles, skin and hair. Because of our bio-individuality, protein requirements vary dramatically from person to person. I recommend experimenting with reducing or increasing your amount of protein intake, trying different sources and listening to your body to find out what is best for your individual dietary needs at this point in time. The majority of Americans today eat way too much protein, but for some people, especially O blood types and men, eating a protein-rich food only once a day may be inadequate. Low protein can lead to low energy and all kinds of cravings.

On the other end, many people feel lighter, clearer and a lessening of disease symptoms when they reduce animal food. Animal foods are rich in fat and cholesterol. Disorders such as heart disease, cancer, overweight, obesity and high blood pressure can all be linked to an excess of animal foods. Other health concerns that can clear up when people reduce animal protein are constipation, low energy, body odor and sugar cravings. Also, a worldwide meat-based diet is not environmentally sustainable for the planet. For these reasons, I generally recommend reducing animal meat.

The vegan lifestyle is becoming increasingly popular, especially among young people. In addition to not eating any food coming from an animal source—including meat, chicken, eggs and dairy—they strongly prefer not to wear shoes, belts or any other clothing made from an animal source.

Vegetarian and vegan people often attempt to get their protein needs met through beans and bean products. Although beans contain protein, that protein is not easily assimilated. Beans are one of the most difficult foods to digest, and vegetarians must learn to properly prepare their beans to get maximum nutritional benefit and reduce gas and indigestion. Usually, this means choosing smaller beans and cooking them longer than you imagine is necessary.

In Mexico and central America, where beans are a fundamental part of the daily diet, the most frequent bean dish is refried beans. They are cooked once and then refried in oil or butter to ensure simpler digestion. A similar situation exists in Japanese cuisine with soybeans. Rarely, if ever, do the Japanese eat soybeans unless the beans have first been fermented or aged. Then they convert the beans into foods like miso, soy sauce and natto. They also eat tofu in small amounts.

Out of all the beans, soy is the most difficult to digest. After wheat, soy is one of the most common allergens, and people don't realize this because it is labeled as a health food. Remember, just because something is sold in a natural food store does not mean that it's healthy. Many vegetarians and vegans rely on tofu, soy milk (which is really tofu that has not been coagulated) and other soy products as their main source of protein. They pour soy milk on their cereal, have soy smoothies and cook tofu in dinner every night. Tofu is a good source of protein, but I recommend it be eaten in moderate quantity. Not only can it cause allergic reactions and digestive upset, it is also a highly processed food. The exception is edamame, a young, whole soybean that is relatively easy to assimilate.

There is some research showing that a certain chemical found in soy, called genistein, can potentially damage fertility, especially in men. Traditionally, in Zen monasteries, men would eat tofu to help reduce their sex drive so they could sustain a celibate lifestyle. So men, if you want to be celibate, tofu is a great food for you. However, if that is not your mission, you may want to avoid eating too much tofu.

For those who refuse to eat animal meat, eggs may be a good source of protein. High quality yogurt may also be a good option for those who are not lactose intolerant. I strongly encourage buying organic eggs and dairy that are free from hormones and antibiotics.

Many Americans prefer beef as their main source of protein. Including other animal meats—such as duck, pheasant, buffalo, lamb, chicken and fish—and rotating these in your diet helps to avoid the stagnancy and health concerns associated with excess beef consumption, including heart disease, high blood pressure, constipation, high cholesterol and mad cow disease. Quality of meat is really important, and organic is always the best option. Generally, animals on organic farms are treated much more humanely than on factory farms. As I discussed in chapter 2, we take in an animal's energy when we eat it. Wouldn't you rather take in the energy of an animal that was not cruelly treated through its lifetime?

When deciding how much animal food to eat with a meal, I urge you to follow the guidance of Dr. Barry Sears, author of *Enter the Zone* and guest lecturer at our institute, who recommends eating a piece of meat "no bigger and no thicker than the palm of your hand." This is about four ounces per portion, and a much healthier choice than having a huge slab of meat as a main course.

We intuitively know that animal food increases our sense of personal power, self-esteem, confidence and aggressiveness. That's why many people eat excessive amounts and suffer consequences of poor health and life-threatening illness. Those who eat a plant-based diet are likely to be more balanced and healthy, but can become too fixed. Life stops becoming fun because they don't have the energy to go out, hit the town and enjoy themselves. They are more like a plant. They just want to sit still. Look around at what most CEOs, politicians and athletes eat. Not too many vegetarians there! Again, there is no right and wrong here. Food is not religion. There is no special heaven reserved for vegetarians. So please find the fuel that is most suitable for your current needs. Finding the optimum protein intake is a key to balanced energy, as well as emotional and mental well-being.

• • • 7. Less Meat, Dairy, Sugar, Chemicalized Artificial Junk Foods; Less Coffee, Alcohol and Tobacco • • •

I would rather add than take away from any individual's diet. However, most people who reduce these elements in their daily diet feel more energized and, if sick, are better able to recover their health and vitality. The effects of consuming too much dairy, sugar and coffee are covered in chapter 8. The impact of smoking and drinking on the body is well known, and could fill an entire book of its own.

• • • 8. Develop Easy and Reliable Ways to Nurture Your Body • • •

The hot water bottle and tongue scraper—all discussed in earlier chapters—are tools you can use daily to create a loving relationship with your body. The hot towel scrub, described in detail in the Exercises section of this chapter, is an incredible tool for relaxation, circulation and detoxification. If you use it a few minutes every day, or even once a week, your body will thank you. Similarly, the hot water bottle takes just a minute to fill, and is a powerful implement to relieve stress and digestive pain, or heat up a cold bed at night. The tongue scraper takes just seconds to use, and can easily be worked into your morning and nighttime rituals. It removes the gunk from your tongue, thereby making your food more flavorful. It reduces cravings because your clean tongue has less food memories on its tip. In India, it is believed to improve enunciation, that a polished tongue refines your speaking. And it's praised by dentists for reducing bacteria in the mouth. These are three of the fastest, easiest and least expensive means of creating a new level of health.

• • • 9. Have Healthy Relationships That Support You • • •

The first people we relate with are members of our birth family. Connecting with these people—with mothers, fathers, siblings, aunts, uncles, grandparents—is challenging for some. I encourage you to learn how to be on good terms with them, if you are not already, without compromising yourself. The same goes true with the family you create—with spouses, children and in-laws.

It's rare that I meet someone who feels entirely supported by their family, friends, coworkers, boss and significant other. Sometimes the answer to getting the support you need is as simple as asking for help from these people, or from a professional. Other times, the answer may lie in creating new relationships and letting go of the old ones that no longer serve you.

Figuring out what kind of love relationship works best for you is crucial. For many, a happy marriage made early is their main goal. They are clear that they want to have children, build a firm structure for their whole life and for future generations. Others look for alternatives to marriage or look to marry later in life. It is important that you take time to determine what you want, and then work practically and positively towards bringing it into being. Having a dream is one thing. Making it happen is another. And again, don't hesitate to ask for help with this if you need it.

• • • 10. Find Physical Activity You Enjoy and Do It Regularly • • •

A lot of people go to great lengths to make sure they are eating healthy food, while not exercising sufficiently. They don't seem to realize that movement aids digestion, assimilation, circulation and respiration.

Many people don't like exercising. It's challenging for them to find an exercise they enjoy. Think about what you loved to do as a kid. Did you dance or bike or hike? This is a good place to start when looking for a new exercise routine. Maybe there is a gym or yoga studio near your home or on the way to the office where you can go and work out. It's important to find a location that's convenient, and where the atmosphere is pleasant, comfortable and welcoming. This will enhance your chances of going regularly.

There is a great difference between exercising indoors and outdoors. Part of exercising can be about reconnecting with nature, perhaps going to a large park if you are a city dweller. Getting out to a rural environment—somewhere you can breathe clean, fresh air, hear the birds and see the sky—on a regular basis can be very helpful. We can live without food for months, and without water for days, but we cannot live without air for more than a few minutes, so it makes sense that air quality is essential to life quality.

• • • 11. Find Work You Love or a Way to Love the Work You Have • • •

Career can often be one of the most dysfunctional areas of life. Many adults resign themselves to doing tedious work in jobs, offices and corporations that are not in alignment with who they are. And they do this not for a day, a week or a month, but for years and decades. Sometimes they are working in fields that are diametrically opposed to their own personal values. As a long-term lifestyle, this is bound to affect their health. If you are one of these people, I encourage you to be more courageous and proactive in remedying the situation. Do you believe we are spiritual beings in a material world? If so, I think you'll agree that what we do all day, every day is central to why we are here.

Many people feel trapped in jobs because they have a retirement fund, 401K plan or accrued benefits. They know they should leave, but they have a mortgage or bills to pay, and they just need to work a few more years before they can quit or retire. If this describes you, the challenge is to find a way to love the work you do. This might mean making your office environment more attractive, identifying people at work who can be allies and avoiding people who are irritating. Get an office with a nice view if you can, use a comfortable chair that supports your back and take stretch breaks every hour.

• • • 12. Develop a Spiritual Practice • • •

Spirituality is what gives depth and meaning to life, creating the feeling of divine order and harmony that exists above and beyond human limitations. For some, this means embracing their religion of birth, following the traditions of their ancestors and seeking depth through prayer and with God. Others feel discontented with their past and explore new avenues, such as Eastern religions, meditation or the religion of their partner. For people who are agnostic or atheist, being spiritual may mean going for a walk in the late evening and feeling the vastness of the night sky with all its stars, or walking in the mountains or by the ocean and enjoying the sense of infinite, endless space. It has been my experience that when people feel connected with the big picture, they get healthier faster.

exercises

1. Your First Step

Choose one of the 12 steps. What is your first step? (#4) less meat, dairy, sugar, coffee, alcahol, chemi junds food

Do only this one for one week.

What are three things you can do to support yourself in making this happen over the next week?

1. Have tea instead of coffee

2. Cook delicious whole foods

3. Use natural sugars such as fruits or sweet vegies instead of prosessed refined sugar

Great—now go and do them!

Check back in with yourself after one week. How did it go? What worked and what didn't? Are you ready to add another step? If so, pick the next one that resonates with you. If not, focus on maintaining the first step until you are ready to add the next. Continue this process until you are doing all 12 steps. Go at your own pace. You will see and feel the difference in your body, mind and spirit.

2. Hot Towel Scrub

The skin is the body's largest organ of elimination. More dead cells, toxins and waste products from the body get eliminated through the skin than through urinating and defecating. Stimulating the pores of your skin with a rubbing action allows them to eliminate better. The only thing separating you from your external environment is your skin. The hot towel scrub rejuvenates this living organ, creating a better two-way flow of sensory information between you and your environment. It is a great source of primary food because it creates a loving connection between you and your body. Also, the heat and friction helps to melt away subcutaneous fat and break down cellulite.

Take a wash cloth, dip it into hot water or hold it under running hot water, wring it out, and then rub your entire body for five to 10 minutes. There is no right direction in which to rub—head to toe, toe to head, towards the heart, away from the heart, whatever feels easy and natural for you. It's invigorating and refreshing if you do it in the morning, calming and relaxing if you do it in the evening after work or at night before you go to bed. It has a neutralizing and balancing effect on the mind.

Some people say it's similar to using a loofah or skin brush, but the added effect of using heat to open pores and break down fat is very important, so don't settle for brushing. Also, take the trouble not to do this in the shower. Instead, stand by a sink. It makes a difference because showering is such a routine, mechanical act. By the sink, you are looking in the mirror, seeing your body, and you are more present to the sensations the hot towel scrub is creating in you.

When I show a wash cloth to my students and say, "This will change your life," they are naturally skeptical. But afterwards I get much positive feedback, like, "I can't believe how well this works!" and "I feel my skin opening up, vibrating," and "I've fallen in love with my body."

Try it.

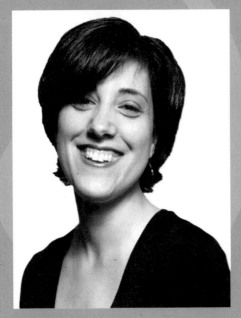

In November 1992 I was diagnosed with multiple sclerosis. I was put on many synthetic drugs and began gaining a lot of weight. In spite of the meds, my health remained poor. I began researching alternative medicine and holistic therapies, and after changing my diet to whole and natural foods, I was able to lose weight, gain my strength back and feel like myself again. By 1997 my health had dramatically improved.

After my recovery, I became the go-to person among my friends and family for dietary advice. Yet, oddly enough, they rarely took my advice. I often felt alone because most of my friends, family and coworkers were not interested in a holistic viewpoint.

When a coworker handed me a brochure for Integrative Nutrition, I immediately enrolled. During my school year, I realized that I had been a preacher of good health, rather than an effective teacher. I learned how to listen to people, gained confidence and committed myself to supporting other parents and children with their health and nutrition needs.

In November 2003 I founded Nourish Our Kids, Inc. Nourish Our Kids is dedicated to educating parents and their children on ways to maintain a natural and healthy diet and lifestyle. Since 2003, along with the Children's Aid Society, I have personally been involved in creating and deploying an obesity prevention curriculum for preschoolers in three health start schools located in NYC. Nourish Our Kids has also conducted several on-site diet, health and fitness programs with adolescents in after-school centers. In the near future, Nourish Our Kids has plans to launch a series of national programs for preschoolers and their parents.

Donna Terjesen
Forest Hills, NY
Graduate 2001
www.nourishourkids.com

The school gave me the credentials and the self-assurance I needed to create a business that makes a difference. Integrative Nutrition empowers everyone who enrolls to choose their own path and to create a life they love.

chapter 8

No foods are forbidden
except when your body tells you so.
Lima Ohsawa

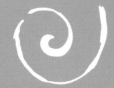

foods to avoid or minimize

B Y NOW YOU HAVE GRASPED THE
fundamentals of maintaining a healthy diet. In spite of the enormous amount of confusing and often
contradictory information that regularly floods the world of nutrition and health, the basics are simple.
Most people need less meat, milk, sugar, chemicalized artificial junk food, alcohol, caffeine and tobacco.
They need to eat more whole grains and vegetables, especially greens, and drink more water.

I want to emphasize, however, that no food is innately bad. If you really want to have some fried
chicken, a burger, a chocolate chip cookie or ice cream, it's okay within the overall context of a healthy
diet. I am not in favor of fanaticism or extreme food practices. As I said before, it's not what you eat some
of the time, it's what you eat most of the time that makes a difference.

In this chapter, we take a closer look at some extreme foods so that you can have a clearer understanding of their effects. We'll start with the most challenging of all: sugar.

• • • Sugar • • •

The first sugar refinery in the U.S. was built in 1689. Its product was very popular. Colonists soon began
to sweeten their breakfast porridge with refined sugar, and within 10 years individual consumption had
reached four pounds a year. Current estimates show that 150 pounds of sugar are now consumed each
year, per person, on average.

Sugar qualifies as an addictive substance for two reasons:
1) Eating even a small amount creates a desire for more.
2) Suddenly quitting causes withdrawal symptoms such as headaches, mood swings, cravings and fatigue.

Sugar is a simple carbohydrate that occurs naturally in foods such as grains, beans, vegetables and fruit. When unprocessed, it is linked with all kinds of vitamins, minerals, enzymes and proteins. When brown rice or other whole grain is cooked, chewed and digested, the natural carbohydrates break down uniformly into separate glucose molecules. These enter the bloodstream, where they are burned smoothly and evenly, and all the good stuff can be absorbed.

Refined table sugar, called sucrose, is very different. Extracted from either cane or beet, it requires extra effort from the body to digest because it lacks vitamins, minerals and fiber. The body must deplete its own store of minerals and enzymes to absorb sucrose properly. Therefore, instead of providing the body with nutrition, it results in deficiency. It enters swiftly into the bloodstream and wreaks havoc on the blood sugar level, first pushing it sky-high—causing excitability, nervous tension and hyperactivity—then dropping it extremely low—causing fatigue, depression, weariness and exhaustion. These days, health-conscious people know their blood sugar levels go up and down on a sugar-induced high, but they often don't realize the emotional roller coaster ride that accompanies this. We feel happy and energetic for a while and then suddenly, unexplainably, we find ourselves arguing with our friend or lover.

Today sugar is in children's cereals, cakes, cookies and desserts, and also in canned vegetables, baby food, bread and tomato sauce. It is often disguised in fancy language, labeled corn syrup, dextrose, maltose, glucose or fructose. Overconsumption of these refined sweets has led to an explosion of hypoglycemia and type 2 diabetes.

Much of the U.S. population is hypoglycemic. Hypoglycemia literally means "low glucose levels in the blood." Glucose is a type of sugar that provides energy to every cell in the body. Our bodies normally maintain blood glucose levels within a narrow range. When this homeostasis is lost, hypoglycemia can result. A poor diet, especially an excess of refined sugars, can cause a gradual breakdown in our body's ability to manage blood glucose. When this happens, blood glucose levels may initially spike after a meal (hyperglycemia) and then crash to abnormally low levels several hours after the meal (hypoglycemia). This roller-coaster effect is thought to instigate type 2 diabetes. It may take years for hypoglycemia to develop into full-blown diabetes, but the sooner you intervene the better. Symptoms of hypoglycemia include faintness, dizziness, sweating, anxiety and hunger. If you think you have hypoglycemia, you definitely want to reduce the amount of refined sugar in your diet.

Diabetes is the sixth leading cause of death in the U.S., and growing. Type 1 diabetes, known as juvenile onset or insulin-dependent diabetes, typically develops in childhood or early adulthood. With type 1 diabetes, the pancreas is unable to produce insulin. When a person without diabetes eats something that creates glucose in the blood, the pancreas produces insulin in order to maintain blood sugar balance. Insulin acts as the gatekeeper, allowing the proper amount of glucose into the body's cells to be utilized as fuel. People with type 1 diabetes must rely on daily injections of insulin to keep their blood sugar from getting too high.

Type 2 diabetes usually develops much later in life, though recently it is on the rise in children and adolescents. With type 2 diabetes, the pancreas is still capable of producing insulin, but the cells in the body are less responsive to it. Of the two types of diabetes, type 2 is by far the most prevalent. One of the most alarming statistics in medicine right now is the rate at which Americans are being stricken with this form of diabetes. This is heartbreaking because it can be prevented by reducing processed sugar and eating a healthy, balanced diet.

When people lose the ability to sustain a proper blood sugar level, the entire human organism is affected. The healthy body exists in a state of homeostasis, maintaining a steady balance within all systems that ensures smooth functioning for the entire being. Take body temperature for example. Somehow the body knows how to maintain a steady temperature of 98.6 degrees. If it gets overheated, it perspires to cool us down; if it gets too cold, it shivers to warm us up. There are many systems like this in the body. It knows when to urinate; otherwise your bladder would swell and explode. It knows when to go to sleep; otherwise, you could drift into slumber while driving and crash. These are systems the body maintains by itself, for itself, without any need to be consciously controlled or reminded, and they are all interlinked. Because blood sugar is part of the hormonal system and thereby interconnected with many vital body control systems—including the sexual reproductive system, adrenal glands, thyroid and pineal glands—the breakdown of blood sugar regulation can lead to the breakdown of another system, and another until the entire organism is out of whack.

But sugar isn't the problem. The problem is the vicious, addictive cycle we have created by eating processed sugar, feeling the rush, crashing, and then taking in more sugar to begin the whole mess again. If we are on a healthy, balanced diet, nourishing ourselves with milder forms of sweet, we don't need a big sugar hit from a candy bar or soda to boost our energy level.

Increasingly more people understand the need to find alternatives to sugar, creating a demand that has produced a stream of artificial sweeteners, such as saccharin (Sweet'N Low) and aspartame (Equal, NutraSweet). Unfortunately, these products have been linked to serious health problems, but as public demand increases, more options are continually being explored. Sucralose is one of the latest to hit the market, and under the brand name Splenda it has become the nation's number one selling artificial sweetener in a remarkably short period of time. Sucralose is made from sugar in a patented five-step process that substitutes three atoms of chlorine for three of hydrogen-oxygen, converting sugar into a fructo-galactose molecule. This type of molecule does not occur in nature, and therefore your body does not possess the ability to properly metabolize it. So although sucralose tastes like sugar and sweetens like sugar, it is not assimilated by the body. This is why it has zero calories. Questions about the safety of sucralose are already being raised, but it's too early to say what the negative effects are. One can assume it would not enhance health.

From a holistic point of view, it makes more sense to go with naturally occurring sweeteners, rather than artificial products. However, switching from white to brown sugar or coarse turbinado sugar is not the answer. These alternatives contain 96% sucrose, not much of an improvement on the 99.9% sucrose content in refined white sugar.

Here are some better options:

Agave Nectar

Agave nectar is a natural sweetener made from the juice of the agave cactus. It is approximately 1.4 times sweeter than refined sugar, but does not create a "sugar rush," and is less disturbing to the body's blood sugar levels.

Barley Malt

Barley malt is created when fermenting bacteria in barley turns its starch into sugars, mostly maltose. The final product is more of a "whole food" than some other sweeteners. It's not as sweet as sugar, so you may need to add up to 50% more in recipes.

Brown Rice Syrup

Consists of brown rice that has been ground, cooked and mixed with enzymes that change the starch into maltose. Brown rice syrup tastes like moderately sweet butterscotch and can be quite delicious. In recipes, you may have to use up to 50% more brown rice syrup than sugar, while reducing the amount of other liquids.

Date Sugar

Date sugar is not a sugar, but rather finely ground dates containing all of the fruit's nutrients and minerals. If you like the taste of dates, this will definitely appeal to you. Date sugar can be used as a direct replacement for sugar. While quite sweet, date sugar will not impart a sugary taste to cooked dishes.

Honey

One of the oldest natural sweeteners, honey is sweeter than sugar, with different flavors depending on plant source. Some honeys are dark and strongly flavored. Raw honey contains small amounts of enzymes, minerals and vitamins.

Maple Syrup

Maple syrup adds a nice flavor to foods. Make sure you buy 100% pure maple syrup, not maple-flavored corn syrup. Organic varieties are best.

Molasses

Organic molasses is probably the most nutritious sweetener derived from sugar cane. Different types of molasses have different flavors, but most of them impart a very distinctive taste. Use less molasses than you would sugar. Sucanat is a brand name for an organic evaporated cane juice product that has been blended with organic molasses, and is 88% sucrose, with fructose and dextrose. It can be used like white sugar, but retains more of the vitamins and minerals of sugar cane.

Stevia

Stevia is an herb from the rain forests of the Amazon that has been used for centuries by native South Americans. The extract from stevia leaves is said to be 100 to 300 times sweeter than white sugar, and can be used in cooking and baking as well as in drinks. Stevia extract does not affect blood sugar levels and has zero calories. Stevia is available in a powder or liquid in most natural food stores. Be sure to get the green or brown liquids or powders though, because the white and clear versions are highly refined, lack nutrients and can lead to imbalance.

• • • Dairy • • •

Females of all mammalian species in the wild nourish their babies with their own milk and stop after a relatively brief period of growth. After this time, young mammals never again show any interest in milk, nor do they have access to it. Humans are the only mammals who do not follow this system.

I am not saying we should stop enjoying the wide range of dairy products available in modern society, but it is worth acknowledging the plain truth: We don't need dairy. It is not an essential part of diet, and most adults around the world do not consume it. In fact, most of them can't because they are lactose intolerant, a term used for people whose digestive systems lack the enzymes needed to digest dairy.

Even those who can digest dairy typically consume too much. Dairy products, especially cheese and ice cream, are loaded with fat and cholesterol that contribute to clogged arteries and heart disease. In addition, dairy has been cited as a significant cause in the following ailments: women's menstrual pains, asthma, brain fog, mucus, and a wide range of allergies with symptoms such as skin conditions and mood swings. Many people never know their problems are caused by dairy sensitivity, taking various medications instead. A brief break from dairy often leads to surprising improvements in many health conditions.

There's also concern about the use of bovine growth hormone, or BST, a controversial, genetically engineered growth hormone that increases milk production in cows. The manufacturers of BST have claimed for years that this hormone has no adverse side effects on animals or humans, but many people disagree and it has been banned in some countries, including Canada.

Some research has shown that a cow's natural hormones have an even more serious effect than BST on the health of women in this country. Dr. Walter Willett, head of nutrition at Harvard, is concerned that there may be a link between the high rate of breast cancer among American women and the fact that, in order to maximize milk production, cows are now kept pregnant most of the time on both commercial and organic farms. During pregnancy female cows' hormones like estrogen and progesterone go sky-high, and these hormones are present in their milk. It is this high hormone content that Dr. Willett connects to human cancer of the breast. Assuming Dr. Willett's concerns about breast cancer are justified, I do suggest that women who regularly consume significant amounts of dairy products consider seeking alternatives, or at the very least take care to improve the quality and reduce the quantity of dairy they are eating.

If you eat dairy, I strongly encourage eating organic, although even organic dairies can be controversial. Horizon Organic Dairy, the largest supplier of organic milk in the U.S. and owned by the largest processor and distributor of milk in the U.S., has recently been questioned for not enforcing the criteria necessary to be labeled organic. On genuine organic dairy farms, cows are raised on open pastures, fed grass and not given extra hormones. Experts say the cows at Horizon are raised in pens and fed mostly protein and grains. Although the milk from the Horizon farms may not be the best possible quality, it is better than the milk produced from dairy factories, with thousands of cows pumped up with antibiotics and confined in small spaces. Organic milk costs up to twice as much as regular milk, but I contend that it is worth it. Just make sure you are educated about its source.

Contrary to popular belief, dairy does not stop osteoporosis or bone fracture in the elderly by boosting calcium intake. In fact, numerous studies demonstrate that countries with the highest intake of dairy, such as the U.S. and Holland, have the highest incidence of osteoporosis and fractures, while countries with the lowest dairy intake, such as Japan and South Africa, have the lowest rates of osteoporosis and fracture. Healthy bones need calcium, magnesium, phosphorus, boron, copper, manganese, zinc and many vitamins. An excess of calcium without these other vitamins and minerals can actually increase the likelihood of fracture. Vegetable foods high in calcium, such as collards, bok choy and sea vegetables, also contain an abundance of magnesium and other minerals, unlike milk products, which have an overabundance of calcium. Eating a good amount of green vegetables, whole grains and sea vegetables can provide all the essential calcium needed for the human body, without the added negative side effects of dairy.

For some people, dairy is an emotional issue. It's a food that provokes a lot of feelings and attachment. From a psychological point of view, this could be attributed to the nourishing memories of breast-feeding. When I point out the hazards of high dairy consumption in the school, many students are adamant in their refusal to give it up. If you have an emotional response to the idea of reducing or eliminating dairy, it may be helpful to examine the source of these emotions. Perhaps dairy is providing you with nourishment outside of the protein, fat and minerals, nourishment that is not about secondary food nutrition. If so, try to think of other ways you can get this nourishment.

• • • Meat • • •

We are being inundated every day with messages—whether from advertising or the pages of the latest high protein diet book—emphasizing the need to eat more and more meat. This is dangerous. Excessive meat eating is clearly implicated in heart disease, several types of cancer (especially colon cancer) and the common problem of constipation.

Men particularly don't like it when I talk about the need to eat less meat, but it still needs to be said. So let me get to the bottom line. Any kind of mass-produced, factory-farmed, commercially grown meat—whether it is beef, pork or chicken—is loaded with hormones and antibiotics that are designed to generate the maximum amount of meat per animal, and therefore the maximum amount of profit for the producers. When you eat the meat, you eat the hormones and antibiotics.

Red meat, especially, is full of saturated fats, has no fiber and no phytochemicals. Commercially raised chickens are not a good alternative, as they have been found to contain excessive levels of antibiotics, steroids and growth hormones. Moreover, the fat levels of commercially raised chickens are over three times the level of their free-range relatives.

Remember, too, that these animals suffer, and this suffering is passed on to those who consume their meat. We've already discussed how humans take on the qualities of animals we consume through cross-species transference, and we also take on their pain of being reared in cruel conditions.

For many people, eating meat is a question of ethics. Some vegetarians and vegans are adamant in their belief that eating animals is inhumane. Other people feel as strongly about their need to eat meat. I simply believe people should choose whatever protein source feels comfortable for them. I pray for the day when all people can thrive on a vegetarian diet. But through my years of experience, I have seen many vegetarian-type people become healthier by incorporating small amounts of organic meat into their diet. I have also seen many heavy meat eaters become healthier when reducing the amount of meat in their diet.

A funny thing happens to the students at our school. The ones who come in as heavy meat eaters always graduate with a more vegetarian-type diet, and many who enroll as vegans or vegetarians leave as fish or meat eaters. This shows that people can learn how to find balance in their individual needs for protein.

Keep in mind that, according to Dr. Peter D'Adamo, the digestive systems of people with O blood type are more suited to absorbing meat than other types. And if you come from a meat-eating culture, it makes more sense for you to be including meat in your diet than if you are from a long line of vegetarians in the Philippines.

Bearing all this in mind, I generally recommend people limit meat eating to a few times a week, and supplement this with other protein sources such as eggs, beans, tofu and whole grains. If you are a regular meat eater, choose organic meats whenever possible.

• • • Coffee • • •

Millions of Americans jump-start their day with a cup of coffee, and then drink another cup halfway through the morning. Not surprisingly, coffee represents 75% of all caffeine consumed in the U.S. And if sugar is America's number one addiction, then coffee ranks a very close second. Caffeine is a drug, and we are a nation of drug users.

Drinking coffee isn't just a matter of personal taste. It's become a cultural habit, an entertainment and a form of comfort. It's warm, it's foamy, and it tastes good with sugar, chocolate powder or cinnamon on top. It's an enjoyable social moment, a ritual and a symbol of dynamic, busy, working people.

A lot of time and money has been spent by coffee producers to reassure the American public that drinking coffee isn't bad for health, including a general statement that up to three cups per day causes no health problems whatsoever. Caffeine, the essential ingredient, is said to enhance alertness, concentration and mental and physical performance, and its negative side effects are downplayed.

Coffee is, essentially, an adrenalin delivery system that jolts the body's central nervous system. In the short term, this jolting action wakes us up, gets us going. In the long term, the constant and unnatural stimulation of our nerves creates stress levels that damage the resilience of the immune system, which protects against disease. Coffee is part of a stress cycle: We need coffee to keep up the pace, and coffee itself helps to create the nervous energy of this pace.

Caffeine should be given up slowly. Caffeine withdrawal is not fun, and people often report headaches and mood swings. I recommend quitting by slowly reducing the number of cups of coffee you drink each day, or by diluting full-strength coffee with decaffeinated. Crowd out coffee by frequently drinking bottled or filtered water throughout the day. Rediscover the delights of drinking tea. Green tea contains a much milder amount of caffeine and can be a great way to get over the withdrawal headaches.

• • • Salt • • •

Most medical experts agree that diets high in sodium are a major cause of high blood pressure as well as pre-hypertension. High blood pressure and pre-hypertension significantly increase the risk of having a heart attack or stroke. Today roughly 65 million Americans have high blood pressure and another 45 million have pre-hypertension, and while excessive salt intake is not the only cause of these alarming statistics, it is a contributing factor.

Restaurant foods, fast foods and processed, packaged junk foods contribute the majority of sodium to our diets. Campaigners for more public awareness about the dangers of excessive salt consumption claim that if we could reduce the sodium in processed and restaurant foods by half, we could save thousands of lives. My solution is more simple and immediate: Master the art of home cooking and you will solve the problem.

I strongly recommend using a high quality sea salt for home cooking. There is a huge difference between high quality, natural sea salt and poor quality, refined table salt. For the most part, people today use processed, sparkling white salt that is stripped of the trace elements and minerals in high quality sea salt. Food companies also put additives—such as sugar and potassium iodide—into refined salt. Potassium iodine is added to avoid iron deficiency and thyroid disease, but it has actually been linked to the recent increase in hyperthyroidism among Americans. All this processing takes place to make salt less expensive and a prettier color, as natural sea salt has a brownish tint.

Throughout history, people have used salt to season food and as a natural preservative. Salt is not bad. In fact, good quality sea salt can contain up to 92 minerals. The health problems associated with over-consumption of salt are from the refined, processed, white sparkly salt that is in prepared foods and that so many Americans use at home. Using high quality sea salt in limited quantities is a healthier and tastier way to get minerals and satisfy your body's cravings for salty flavor.

• • • Chocolate • • •

Eating healthy doesn't only mean cutting back on food. For many of us, being moderate means including more of a food that we may have limited because we thought it was bad. The good news is chocolate is the ideal example, and certainly worthy of praise. Long regarded as a sinful, addictive and fattening temptation, chocolate can be a health-promoting food and provide a natural feel-good high. Chocolate comes to us courtesy of the cacao plant, which literally means "food of the gods." Cacao is high in iron, calcium, potassium and vitamins A, B, C and D. It can also provide protection against cancer, heart disease and high blood pressure. One of the reasons chocolate has a bad rap is because most chocolate sold in supermarkets and convenient stores has high amounts of added sugar, fat and trans fats. For this reason, I recommend finding an organic brand with a high percentage of cacao. In a world that is becoming increasingly contracted and stressful, chocolate gives people a sense of lightness, expansiveness, comfort and relaxation.

exercises

1. Reduce One Food

Choose one food from this chapter—sugar, dairy, meat, coffee or salt—that you feel would be useful to reduce.

Which one is it? _Sugar_

For one week, gently decrease your consumption of this one food and write down the results.

What is difficult about reducing this food?

Sugar is everywhere and it's addictive

What is easy about reducing this food?

There are many ^natural substitutes for sugar that I am finding very satisfying.

Does your body feel different? Healthier?

Yes. And I can feel the negative impact immediately when I eat, for example, a very sugary cookie.

Are you going to continue to minimize this food in your diet?

Yes, I believe that the more I continue to minimize sugar in my diet, the more emotionally + physically stable I will feel.

2. Be Bad

Now that I've covered foods that can lead to health problems when overconsumed, I want to introduce you to the joy and freedom of throwing away the rules and being bad. For many of you, being good, returning all phone calls and e-mails, always being on time, being balanced and full of integrity and responsibility is your highest priority.

But you are not perfect. Nobody is. And pretending to be perfect does not serve you or those you know and love. In a way, it is inauthentic to live our lives pretending to be perfect.

I invite you over the next week to do something bad every single day. When I say "bad," I mean something you feel you shouldn't do or feel is irresponsible. Obviously, I'm not asking you to rob a bank or hurt another human being. Perhaps you'll delete unread e-mails, play hooky from work, eat an exotic dessert or tell someone what you really think. Start out slow. Gradually build your "being bad" muscles.

The purpose behind this exercise is to put you back in charge of your life. Many of us feel like being good is what makes us worthwhile. We put pleasing others above pleasing ourselves. Learning to put yourself first and find your voice is priceless. Why not just tell the truth about yourself? If people like you, great. And if they don't, know that you are still a very good person. This way, you remain true to you. There's nothing more health-promoting than that.

Write down three things you want to do this week to practice being bad:

1. _Eat ice cream_
2. _Take a nap instead of doing chores_
3. _Have a spontaneous romantic moment with a handsome man_

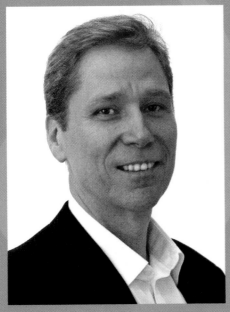

i was searching for tangible information about how to improve my eating and looking for a new career when I found the red magazine for Integrative Nutrition. I immediately knew it was the right place for me. Going to the school was a great experience because I was involved with a community of people who shared my passion for healing the self and being of service to others.

Integrative Nutrition's program left me with a stronger awareness and appreciation for life. My relationships with my wife and son have improved. I really listen to my wife now, and I praise her more, telling her what a great woman she is. My son is 15, and our communication has grown because I no longer try to change him. The best thing I can do is to be an example for him. I feel more present at home and more at ease with myself.

As far as my holistic health counseling business goes, I have had amazing opportunities. Not long ago I met a man who was interested in what I did, so I gave him my card. He became a client, asked me to give a talk at an after-school program he runs, and made me a guest on his live cable TV show that has 150,000 viewers.

Being on TV was really exciting. I could see myself on the screen and I loved it! It's an ethnic cable channel and most of the viewers are from the Indian community in New York. Sugar is seen as an energy booster by many in this community, and there are a lot of heart problems and diabetes as a result. I wanted to get the message out about the harmful effects of sugar and processed foods. The program was called "Secrets of Good Health." I talked about diet and about primary food: the importance of being aware of how our relationships, spirituality, career and physical activity affect our lives. The show was half an hour long and there was supposed to be time for viewers to call in, but the host was so interested in what I was saying that he kept asking questions, and we ran out of time. Several people who saw the show contacted me for health consultations.

Steve Rosenbloom
Graduate 2004
Brooklyn, NY
srose53@earthlink.net

My business is expanding all the time! The work I do as a holistic health counselor is really important. I bring a message to people, it changes their lives, and it changes the world.

Recently, I walked into my boss' office to let him know I was going to India for a month. He looked at me with concern and said, "As long as you're coming back, it's not a problem." "As a matter of fact," I said, "I need to talk to you about this." I told him that once I got back I wanted to reduce my hours so that I could focus more on developing my practice as a holistic health counselor. And he said, "OK. You do a great job. We really want to keep you here." Then he gave me a raise! I couldn't believe it.

Thirteen years ago, I was an active alcoholic. I weighed 220 pounds and my life was in shambles. Today, as a recovered alcoholic, I am healthy, happy and proud to be a holistic health counselor. Joshua Rosenthal and Integrative Nutrition have played a central role in this process.

chapter 9

One cannot think well,
love well, sleep well,
if one has not dined well.

Virginia Woolf

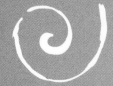

cooking like your life depends on it

TELL PEOPLE TO COOK LIKE THEIR LIFE depends on it because it does. The food we take into our mouth goes into our stomach, where it gets digested and eventually assimilated into the bloodstream. Our blood is what creates our cells, our tissues, our organs, our skin, our hair, our brains and eventually, our thoughts and feelings. We are, at our most basic level, walking food. Learning to cook high quality foods for yourself and those you love can change everything. The three most important aspects of cooking are that the food be homemade, freshly made and lovingly made.

• • • Homemade • • •

Throughout human history, as we have evolved from tribal societies into the extended family and now the nuclear, meals have mostly been eaten together. Not too long ago, dinner was at 6:00 every night, with few exceptions. The meal was made by mom, and the rest of the family members would all come home from work or school, and sit around the table together. The food would be served and everyone would eat while talking about the various events of the day. This ritual bonded people, and the family that ate together, stayed together.

Today everything has changed. People increasingly eat most of their meals out, either in restaurants, delis, fast food places or snacking along the way. Home can be like a hotel, a place only for people to sleep at night. Starting first thing, adults, teenagers and children wake up at different times, go in different directions, eat separately and have little communication throughout the day. By the time dad gets home at night, if there is a dad, the kids are buried deep in their homework, favorite TV shows, video games or Web surfing. It's rare that everyone gets to have a home-cooked meal together. Not only does this schedule create distance in family relationships, but the lack of quality, home-cooked food leads to a deficiency of primary nourishment.

I am a big believer in people eating homemade food as often as possible. As part of this understanding, I'd like to acknowledge the extent to which a woman's traditional work in the home has been undervalued. Whether that work was cooking, keeping the home clean or raising children, all these important jobs are underappreciated in society today. I am not suggesting that women go back to these roles, but it is important to recognize how traditional, motherly nourishment supported the whole family. It kept everyone healthy and happy in many ways.

Cooking for ourselves also has incredible nourishing value. When we put our own energy into the food, we ultimately put that energy back into ourselves. We are nurturing ourselves and our bodies on a variety of levels. When we cook, we have control over the quality and quantity of ingredients we are eating. Our body's natural intelligence will fine-tune our cooking style to have us know just what we need. When we are in a restaurant, we give up that control. We do not know where the food came from, how much salt and spices were added, what kind of oil was used, or the health and cleanliness of the various people who touched our food along the way. By cooking our own food, we ultimately create more love for ourselves, more love for our life, and therefore, more health.

• • • Freshly Made • • •

Food that is fresh affects us differently than the same food that's been sitting out for days. Think about the times you've been in a restaurant and a waiter passes who is carrying a hissing tray of freshly cooked food, piled on a hot, steel plate. There is so much energy coming from that plate that the whole restaurant turns around to see what is happening. We take in that same kind of energy when we eat food that's just been made.

Because of practical convenience, we often eat food that has been canned, frozen, sitting in a freezer or made hours earlier. Sometimes we have to do this, and canned and frozen vegetables can be quite fresh since they're often packaged just after being harvested. Understand that I'm not against eating leftovers. I'm a big fan of cooking once and eating twice, to increase the amount of homemade food in the diet without spending too much time in the kitchen, but I always try to add something fresh to my leftovers. I'll heat them with a little water, olive oil and some fresh herbs, or I'll sauté carrots and onions and add them to my meal. This gives my old food new energy and new flavor.

Getting produce from farm to table is an interesting business. Many fruits and vegetables don't arrive in the store until days after they were harvested, then they sit on the shelf at the store for a few days. Then they spend a few more days in the fridge at home. Not too long ago American food was grown locally. Nowadays most of our food is grown in California. People who live there eat produce that is three to four days fresher than the food people eat on the East Coast. I frequently have the feeling that people I meet from the West Coast are in many ways fresher and more in touch with nature than other Americans. Imagine that for your whole life you had been eating food that was three days fresher than other people's food. It would be bound to have a long-term effect.

In many countries it's common for people to shop for vegetables on the same day they cook them because traditionally they understand the importance of freshness. Most Americans prefer the convenience of shopping only once a week. Wherever you live in America, I would like to point you in the direction of your local farmers' market. The food sold is grown nearby, probably in the same county or at least in the same region or state. It's more alive, and this aliveness will transfer itself to your body.

• • • Lovingly Made • • •

After many years of personal observation, I noticed that food prepared at home by someone who loves us affects us very differently than the exact same food purchased in a restaurant. When we eat our mother's or grandmother's cooking, there is love in the food, there is care in its preparation, there is a different quality and energy. Invisible forces are at work, and they have an alchemical effect on the food itself. It tastes different. It feels different in the body. It affects us differently.

When we eat in a fast food restaurant, the people preparing our food are usually underpaid kitchen workers, living on minimum wage. This fact alone is bound to make the quality of the food we eat very different than home-cooked food. In a restaurant, the managers and cooks are pressured into reducing costs and maximizing profits, and often follow a policy of overflavoring the food with salt, butter and spices so people have more alcohol, or mineral water, or dessert just to balance the strong flavors. There's a totally different set of priorities than someone cooking at home.

I recommend performing a small ritual to increase your awareness of what you are about to do before you cook at home. It could involve something as simple as washing your hands, putting on an apron or taking a moment to close your eyes, take a breath in and set an intention for the meal you are about to create. You may also want to light a candle or put on some music, anything that helps you be more present.

The last few minutes of cooking are usually the most stressful. Everything has to be done at the same time: final flavoring, transferring from cooking pot to serving dish, getting the dining area ready, things like this. It's helpful to have ritual at the end of cooking too, before you dash into the dining room, sit down with your partner, family or guests, and start eating. Here are a couple of suggestions:

1) Pour yourself a glass of water and drink it slowly and meditatively, just to calm down and rehydrate. Cooks tend to become very yang—contracted and single-focused—and this simple act of drinking water will help ease you into a mellower, relaxed state so you can enjoy the meal.
2) Take some of the food and put it on a small plate, smell it and take a moment to appreciate the wonderful things in your life.

After serving the food you've just cooked, resist the temptation to apologize for what's wrong with it. This apologizing is one of the strongest neurotic habits acquired by home cooks. I strongly recommend you do not do this because you will focus your family's attention on the things that you mention, rather than on being grateful for your efforts. You want to have people appreciate you; you want them to think, "Wow! Someone actually took the time to prepare a meal with love for me." If you are proud of your food, your family will enjoy it and appreciate you more, and it will help them remember the value of a homemade, freshly made, lovingly cooked meal.

• • • Simplicity • • •

The main reason people don't cook is because they feel like they don't have the time. It looks too complicated, and they don't know where to start. From the very beginning, they feel overwhelmed. They may open a cookbook and see a recipe for lasagna that looks delicious, but requires many ingredients, with hours of work. So they lose their initial enthusiasm, close the book and forget home cooking. People who find themselves in this situation are confusing taste with function. If you want a fancy, tasty meal, go out to a restaurant. You don't need to be a gourmet chef at home; you need to be able to feed yourself and those you love in a nourishing, convenient way.

Occasionally, you may enjoy making a complex recipe, but for daily diet, you probably want to have simple, down-to-earth meals that can be prepared quickly and easily. It takes under five minutes to prepare a piece of fish or meat, two or three minutes to prepare greens, and then an additional five minutes of cooking time for each. If you decide to make a more complicated meal, most of your ingredients, like grains and vegetables, can come from scratch, but these can be easily complemented with canned or frozen foods. Beans take a long time to cook, so use canned beans. Then you can prepare your whole meal in a few minutes. Cooking simple meals on a regular basis will lead you step by step to a simpler, more relaxed and enjoyable lifestyle.

Home cooking also saves you money. Many people unconsciously spend a lot of money every day on food. People eat most of their meals in cafes, snack bars and restaurants, and this can run to about $30 a day. That's $1,000 a month. Remember, it's expensive to eat out, but inexpensive to eat at home if you do it over a sustained period.

• • • Use a Timer • • •

Just because a recipe takes 40 minutes to cook doesn't mean it takes 40 minutes of your time. Using timers helps you know what's due to be taken off the stove when, and frees you for other activities.

People think that if they make their own food, they have to follow a recipe and be in the kitchen for an hour. This thinking creates a negative attitude. Maybe we don't really have so much else to do, but the idea of waiting around the kitchen seems torturous. Timers allow people to eat in a healthy way without big demands on their schedule.

• • • Burn the Rice • • •

Many people are intimidated by complex ingredients, recipes and cooking time. Please try to keep it simple, allow yourself to experiment and make mistakes. Once you get confident, you will have a lifetime of delicious, home-cooked food for yourself, your family and friends, save thousands of dollars, and increase health, vitality and family relatedness. To reach this desirable goal, you need to understand that there is a learning curve. In the beginning, it will take time, may seem difficult, and you'll likely burn some foods and even some pots. But as you stay with it, cooking will become easier, more enjoyable and hugely rewarding.

• • • Add Flavor • • •

One of the keys to an easy life in the kitchen is to cook food in a simple way, and then make a wide variety of flavorings available so everyone eating can personalize the meal to their own taste. Sometimes, the simplest meals are the most delicious and refreshing. Your best companion in this regard is a condiment tray or "lazy Susan," a circular dish that sits in the middle of the table on a swivel and rotates with the touch of your hand. Fill this with your favorite flavorings. Then people can add the extra flavors they really like to a basic meal. Some love garlic, some love ginger and spices, others prefer more salt, less salt, more oil or less oil. A lazy Susan can hold all of these, plus other standards like nut butters, salsa and salad dressing. People love to personalize their food, and this method makes it much easier for the cook. A list of readily available condiments is at the end of this chapter.

• • • Cook Once, Eat 2 or 3 Times • • •

Whenever you cook, make extra. You don't have to start from scratch at each meal. Take grains as an example. You can cook your favorite grain in the morning and use some for your hot breakfast cereal, perhaps adding some sweet flavor, like fresh fruit or raisins, and something hearty, like tahini or nut butter. Then you can add some different flavor to the leftover grains, or put them into a soup and take it to work for lunch. In the evening, you can add vegetables and protein, and stir-fry the remainder with oil to give it some extra sizzle. If it's green vegetables you're making and you want to save some for later, it's good to run that portion under cold water to stop the cooking process so that they will not be overdone when you go to reheat them. You can also put leftover food into the fridge in small containers for a great, healthy, wholesome snack in between meals. Cooking once and eating two or three times makes you feel like your investments of money on groceries and time in the kitchen were well worth it.

• • • Notice the Effects of Your Cooking • • •

Cooking for yourself is the best way to understand how you are affected by food. Since you know what you are putting into the meal, you can understand its effects on your body and psyche more easily and directly. Maybe you feel sleepy after a meal and want to take a nap, or maybe you feel more active and have the urge to go somewhere and do something in order to generate energy to digest the meal. You will know if your cooking was too much for your body to handle, or if you feel unsatisfied and need more, an extra flavor perhaps or one more ingredient. I encourage you to explore, experiment, and learn to distinguish the foods and quantities that support your health from those that do not.

• • • Cooking with the Seasons • • •

When we buy food at the supermarket, we can get mangoes and bananas in the middle of winter. This is likely not what nature intended. A great way to honor the natural environment in which you live is to look for and use locally grown ingredients. This will help you feel more at home where you are, and more comfortable in yourself. It will also help your body adapt to changes in season. In springtime there are more greens, in summer more fruits and raw foods, in autumn more hardy vegetables and whole grains. In the wintertime you may be drawn to more animal food or richly cooked food. Be aware that during certain times of year when you eat foods that were not meant to be consumed at that particular time, you may become susceptible to colds and flu.

During the summer months, people are out partying, holding barbeques, enjoying outdoor sports, playing on the beach, going on vacation and engaging in other high-energy activities. This is appropriate to the season. With fall, children return to school and people get what I call "squirrelly." Maybe it's a cellular memory from our ancestors who were busy with the harvest season at this time of year that creates the tendency to become busy in September and October, running around, getting ready for winter. Come Halloween, children scour the neighborhood and gather as much sugar and candy as they possibly can. Next come the holidays, and this is when people's actions fall out of pace with what the colder weather should be stimulating in them. At Thanksgiving, Americans nationwide congregate and overeat. The next day everyone complains about how stuffed they are and goes shopping. Then we're into December, with office parties, family get-togethers and social events that usually involve lots of drinking. This leads to Christmas and more overeating, with a final blow-out on New Year's Eve that entails yet more eating and drinking.

All this partying is happening when the normal, natural rhythms of life—colder weather, darker evenings, the end of the growing season—indicate this is the right time to turn inward. Humans are mammals, and mammals have a tendency to hibernate during the winter. They are not really sleeping; they are in a kind of battery saving mode, a state not unlike meditation. But, oddly, Americans do the opposite. Instead of going inward, slowing down and replenishing our energy for springtime, society is set up to keep burning the candle at both ends. Then, in January and February, people feel exhausted, depressed and there is a widespread outbreak of colds and flu. This is mostly people's exhausted immune systems that can not cope with the demands of winter, often combined with the inappropriate food consumption mentioned above.

Doctors have given a special name to the exhaustion and depression experienced during the winter months. They call it "seasonal affective disorder," and many blame it on people not getting enough sunlight. If you have been diagnosed with seasonal affective disorder, I encourage you next fall to experiment and go more slowly, respecting the seasons and eating and drinking moderately. You'll likely feel much different in February; the winter blues will be a thing of the past.

If you want to go to holiday parties, enjoy yourself, but be moderate with food and alcohol, and strive to get enough down time. Remember to home cook with seasonal, locally grown ingredients. Then, if you are not already one of those people who rarely get sick in the wintertime, you will join their ranks. Your immune system will become that strong.

• • • Restaurant Eating • • •

When you have no desire or time to cook, and you find yourself eating in a restaurant, try to be as aware as possible of what you are eating. Say you go into a restaurant and the waiter comes and puts a plate of bread on your table. You may want to ask yourself, before automatically reaching for a roll or slice, "Do I really want to eat this? If I were at home right now, would I eat bread and butter before my meal? What effect does bread have on me?" I know from personal experience that it can feel great to go into a restaurant, sit down and immediately say to the waiter, "Please don't bring any bread to the table."

When you ask the bartender for a menu, and he responds by asking what you'd like to drink, you can ask yourself, "Do I really want a drink? Do I always have a drink when I eat a meal?" Then you can decide whether or not you really want that cocktail.

Regardless of how hungry we are, we often find ourselves at restaurants ordering and eating large quantities of rich and heavy foods that we would never have at home. Most people don't know this, but professional menus are designed for you to choose the most expensive food, or foods that are most profitable for the establishment. As you can see, you need to sharpen your awareness to know clearly what you really want to eat, what you habitually will eat if you don't stop to think about it, and what the restaurant owners would like you to eat.

When eating out, try to keep the menu closed and take a moment to check in with yourself. What do you feel like eating right now? How hungry are you? What are the appropriate foods for you to be eating? The restaurant menu is not designed to answer such questions. It makes food sound so tantalizing, you start thinking, "Oh my God, fudge brownie coated with drizzled chocolate, with a few added twists of sugar-crystallized tangerine, and topped with whipped cream. That sounds incredible." Your mouth is watering so much that you develop complete amnesia, forgetting that you want to be alert and careful about what you are eating instead of being seduced.

Not reading the menu helps in a couple of other ways as well. If you are with friends, enjoying a friendly, social connection, it ensures that you don't all suddenly cut off from each other and bury yourselves in the menus, destroying the convivial atmosphere. It also invites a direct dialogue with the waiter, as you inquire, "What do you recommend that has some vegetables and some protein, either fish or chicken?" When the waiter comes up with a couple of recommendations, you can ask, "What does it come with?"

Keep in mind that restaurants have a lot of vegetables in the kitchen that are not necessarily on the menu. I encourage you to ask the waiter what vegetables are available and if the kitchen can make a side dish of steamed, sautéed vegetables in perhaps olive oil and garlic, or any way you prefer. This will help you get accustomed to building vegetables into all your meals.

• • • Flexitarian • • •

Although I strongly encourage home cooking, I am not saying we must cook all our food or never eat out. It is important to have balance and a flexible attitude. Become a flexitarian. There are times when it is healthier to go to a restaurant rather than stress out about preparing a meal, especially for women who work and have children. During busy times, I encourage eating at restaurants with healthy options and enjoying the food, without guilt. Also, when dining at someone else's house, eating what has been prepared for all the guests can be extremely healthy and healing, even if it is something we would never eat on our own. It can be healthier to just have that piece of pizza, fried chicken or ice cream cake, and not be singled out as the "healthy" one who rejects someone else's food.

Being a health food addict can be isolating. People tend to cook alone, eat alone and feel alienated from society. Sometimes we just want to go out, eat whatever we want and have a great time. And sometimes this can be healthier than staying home alone and eating high quality healthy foods and chewing well. There is a point where people can become overly obsessed with food. This can impede on other important elements of life, including relationships, creativity and just feeling part of. Either we avoid others because we don't want to see what they are eating, or they avoid us because they know we will disapprove of their undisciplined eating habits. We want to have relationships with people as a friend, not as a preacher, and projecting our own food concerns onto others is a great way to lose friends fast. Let others eat as they wish, and learn to accept and enjoy their company, regardless of how many spoons of sugar they stir into their coffee.

exercises

1. Condiment List

Go to the store and pick up a bunch of condiments. Keep them on the table at mealtimes so everyone can flavor and personalize the food to their liking. Getting a lazy Susan to keep on your table and store your condiments on is an option. Here are some condiments that I recommend you try, plus you can add your own favorites:

basic spices
garlic
ginger
turmeric
oregano
cinnamon

peppers
cayenne
chili powder
chili flakes
white pepper
black pepper in a grinder
curry powder

salts
sea salt
gomasio: *grinded sesame seeds with sea salt*

nuts and seeds
tahini
nut butters: *peanut, cashew, almond*
nuts: *pine, brazil, cashews, walnuts, almonds, pistachios*
raw or toasted pumpkin seeds
sunflower seeds
sesame seeds

sweeteners
honey
maple syrup
rice syrup
barley malt

stevia
agave nectar: *natural fructose sweetener*

oils, vinegars, sauces
extra virgin olive oil
toasted sesame oil
coconut oil
chili sesame oil—try Eden brand
umeboshi paste: *a tangy, tart puree made from pickled Japanese plums (umeboshi)*
umeboshi vinegar: *a salty, slightly fruity vinegar; use on grains and vegetables*
balsamic vinegar
apple cider vinegar
Bragg's amino acids
tamari soy sauce
various hot sauces
various salad dressings

sea vegetables
dulse flakes: *sprinkle on soups, salads and vegetables for a rich source of minerals and elements*
nori flakes: *high in protein and dietary fiber; use instead of salt for a slightly nutty, salty taste*

other
nutritional yeast
sprouts: *alfalfa, sunflower, mung*
grated daikon radish
sliced red cabbage
ketchup
mustard

2. Try a New Recipe

Now that you've read all about the benefits of cooking homemade, freshly made, lovingly made food, it is time to try a new recipe. There are many listed in the back of this book, so pick one and cook it for your family or friends. Be sure to get fresh ingredients and to cook with love, thinking about what a pleasure it is to nourish those closest to you.

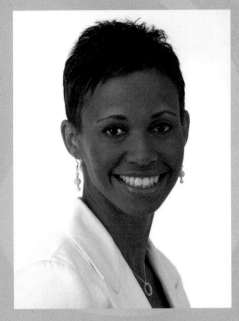

i knew a long time ago that my role in life would be to help people; I just did not know how to make it happen. First, I tried going to law school. After passing the bar and working in various law firms, I quickly realized it was not the type of help I wanted to give. My frustration lead me to the corporate world, where I spent seven years feeling miserable because I knew I was misplaced and not fulfilling my ultimate desire.

Meanwhile, I got married and was blessed with two beautiful children. Working corporate hours and doing what I love—such as cook almost every meal for my family, clean the house and exercise every day—became very challenging. I found myself growing increasingly aware of how keeping physically active, eating high quality food and maintaining a wonderful family life was essential to my health and well-being. In 2004 I saw a graduate from Integrative Nutrition speak at a Black Enterprise Conference, and I decided to enroll in the school.

From the very first day of class, I knew I was in the right place. The energy in the room was incredible, and Joshua's teaching style is definitely off-the-cuff, open, accepting and encouraging. To get to class each weekend, I flew out of the Detroit Airport with three other students who I had met on the school's fabulous Online Community, and we always stayed together at the YMCA. I absolutely loved coming to the city!

The Institute gave me everything I needed to start a business: a website, business cards, a library of books and forms for my clients. More importantly, they instilled in me the belief that I had the innate ability to do what I had always known I was meant to do—help others. The love and support I received from the Integrative Nutrition family, my mentor and classmates is what really got me out there doing this work. Two months after classes began, I quit my six-figure salary job to be a full-time holistic health counselor. I had 15 paying clients in no time at all, and through the money I made from these clients, I paid for my entire education, including travel expenses, before graduation.

Diana Patton
Graduate 2005
Toledo, Ohio
drspatton@buckeye-express.com

I incorporated my business Equilibria, which stands for "Balance for Women," and it is going incredibly well. Currently, I teach sugar education and energy classes, have done a number of paid talks, and conduct presentations for the Women's Nike Canada Basketball Camps. I created "Empowerment Workshops" for young women in colleges in Northwest Ohio, and I am working as a full-time holistic health teacher with a local high school, assisting pregnant teenagers.

Political health issues are very important to me. I have been working on allowing holistic health practitioners to freely practice in the state of Ohio, and on issues related to Ohioans' rights to protest against genetically modified foods and organizations that promote these foods. On the federal level, I am assisting with protecting Americans' rights to clean, healthy food, and to regulate and freely purchase health supplements.

Every day I wake up in love with my life. I have my health; I love my family; I love my career. I know without a doubt that I will continue to be successful as a holistic health counselor and prosperous in body, mind and spirit. The Institute changed my life, and I will tell everyone I meet that it is the best school in the world!

chapter 10

Some people see things as they are and ask, Why?
I dream of things that never were and say, Why not?

People are always blaming their circumstances
for what they are. I don't believe in circumstances.
The people who get on in this world are the people
who get up and look for the circumstances they want,
and if they don't find them, make them.

This is the true joy in life, the being used for a
purpose recognized by yourself as a mighty one;
the being a force of nature instead of a feverish,
selfish little clod of ailments and grievances, complaining that
the world will not devote itself to making you happy.

I am of the opinion that my life belongs to the whole community
and as long as I live, it is my privilege to do for it whatever I can.
I want to be thoroughly used up when I die,
for the harder I work, the more I live.
I rejoice in life for its own sake. Life is no brief candle for me.
It is a sort of splendid torch which I got hold of for the moment,
and I want to make it burn as brightly as possible
before handing it on to future generations.

George Bernard Shaw

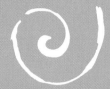

why be healthy?

HEALTH IS A VEHICLE, NOT A destination. There is more to excellent health than just feeling good. Normally, when we are feeling low, dealing with a medical problem or trying to lose weight, we think of health as a goal—something to achieve. Of course, good physical health is an important goal, but if we simply stop there, without exploring further and deeper, we run the risk of missing out on so much more. Robust health allows us to be in the world and achieve things with our life that we wouldn't be able to if we were tired or sick.

Ask yourself, Why be healthy? What would you do with your life if you became healthy? How would you use this gift to enhance your life and the lives of those around you? What would happen if you experienced high-level wellness most of the time? If strength, flexibility, endurance and clear thinking were readily available?

Sadly, most people eat the standard American diet, shop at supermarkets, eat out a majority of the time and graze on packaged snack foods throughout the day. They are increasingly caught up in a matrix mentality concerned with keeping up, fitting in and looking good.

Those who switch to a natural foods diet and lifestyle begin dancing to the beat of a different drummer. We start to think and feel quite differently than others. As our daily diet changes, our blood quality also begins to change. Slowly but surely we begin to notice that we don't fit in like we used to. We naturally see the world from a different perspective than those who are eating fast food and supermarket foods.

As this transition occurs, we may feel like we are on the periphery of society, looking in. And we may be inclined to disguise how differently we feel from others. Many of us develop chameleon-like behavior that allows us to fit into a wide range of environments without standing out. As this trend develops, we may look around, scratch our head and wonder, Why me? Why am I so unusual? Why am I so unlike my brothers and sisters, parents and neighbors?

Some people attribute all this to the idea that we are spiritual beings in a material world. Each of us comes to earth with a different agenda. And for some of us, our path is focused on personal growth and development, which leads to an innate curiosity about food, diet and lifestyle. As we get older, we continually make choices that individuate ourselves from those around us and keep us on track with our destiny.

If that's the case, there's very little value in trying to fit in. Rather than pretending that we are like everyone else, we might as well just take a deep breath, be authentic and be ourselves. There's nothing to be ashamed of.

In my experience, natural food eaters tend to be smarter, healthier, clearer and more in touch with themselves and the natural rhythms of life than people who are eating junk food. It's kind of obvious. And so, we have the potential to step out and create change in the world.

To aid in this process, it's important for us to shift away from the fitting-in mentality. If we continue to expend large amounts of our energy and intelligence just to fit in, we'll have less strength available to focus on the more important aspects of life. We will also be more likely to create health problems for ourselves because we are not openly expressing ourselves. We are hiding our inner light, concealing our unique beauty and shying away from our deeper destiny.

• • • Authentic Self-Expression • • •

As our diet and lifestyle continue to improve, we feel a greater sense of balance, and through this process we become more fully present. We are more likely to notice our breath, feel the breeze on our face and really listen to what people around us are saying. We are more fresh and alert to new situations, with access to a wider choice of behaviors at any given moment. This makes us more likely to steer away from foods and people that are detrimental to our health.

This shows that our personality is not fixed or rigid. The more we slow down and understand ourselves, the more flexible and present we are able to be. Authentic self-expression means being the person we truly are at this point in time. Too many people live life based on events that happened a long time ago: a difficult relationship with a parent, an awkward situation while at school, or a challenging relationship that ended in a strange and unsatisfying way. Many others live life as though they are constantly in preparation for something in the future, blindsighted to the beauty of the moment.

The past is over. The future never arrives. So all you have is the present. The present is a gift, yours to treasure every moment, every day, in every way. You may have had a difficult childhood, challenges with your parents, and all kinds of things that happened to you that never should have happened. But that was then and this is now. And today you are an adult who has a wonderful life. I urge you to let go of the past, forgive it, and know that in some magnificent way, whatever happened was meant to happen. It is exactly those events that have made you who you are today.

• • • Unpredictable Futures • • •

Everyone has a predictable future, a future that would automatically occur by continuing to fit in, following the rules and moving along in life the expected way. In my experience, people avoiding supermarket foods and chemicalized artificial junk foods, who adopt a well-balanced diet and lifestyle, develop a higher degree of creativity, flexibility and aliveness. They are more able to step away from their limited, predictable future and move in unexpected directions that family and friends often find odd, unwise and threatening.

Avoiding junk reduces brain fog and allows people to see opportunities that others can't. It's like when an animal realizes the electrical fence isn't working; suddenly a world of new options opens and all types of unimaginable things become possible. Natural food eaters have a freedom and openness that most people can't fully understand.

It's a powerful experience to know we are strong enough and clear enough to survive and thrive through major lifestyle changes. We develop the capacity and curiosity to start fresh, to explore more creative careers, begin a new relationship, relocate to another area or travel to distant lands. It's our life, and doors of opportunity are opening and closing at every moment.

It's okay to take risks. The world is a safe place. The more we live in balance, respect nature and ourselves, the more likely we will be in the right place at the right time, all the time. The type of relationship we truly want and a career that is in alignment with our deepest values is going to happen, but not without risk, not without our true self-expression. I invite you to tap into and create your unpredictable future.

• • • Spiritual Beings • • •

As you eat more intelligently, you stop medicating yourself, unconsciously using extreme foods as mood-altering drugs. As you stop eating extreme foods that bounce you around on a pinball diet, you naturally become more still. And as you become more centered, you are bound to become clearer, which includes disentangling yourself from the mundane attitudes that were fed to you by the school system, society and the media. The body has to work less hard to maintain homeostasis: blood sugar, temperature and heartbeat are all at optimum levels. When our bodies slow down, we slow down. When we slow down, we increasingly come to experience that there is nothing to do and nowhere to go—that life is just perfectly okay the way that it is.

Despite this beautiful experience, you may find yourself noticing that most people are operating from a confused state, constantly looking for things outside of themselves to fill the void. You may be tempted to fall into self-doubt and try to blend in, throwing yourself back into constant movement and grasping for externals to make yourself feel good since that's what everyone else is doing.

I understand the enjoyment and familiarity of being occupied. After all, I've invested a great deal of time in the development of Integrative Nutrition, so I am well aware of the need to use one's creative energies and be active in the world. But remember that you are a spiritual being in a material world. This is your essential reality, and nothing you achieve or possess on a material level is ever going to fulfill you for long.

Please don't be in a hurry to dismiss or disturb the clear spaces when they come. When the tranquility hits, try to notice and resist the temptation to overeat, argue or busy yourself for the sake of being busy. Allow yourself to live in this relaxed, unoccupied dimension of your being. Give it space. You are a human being, not a human doing. Enjoy the luxury of non-doing. It is an essential part of nature.

• • • Building Your Future • • •

As you learn to nurture yourself, create a new level of health and a fulfilling personal life, space opens up for you to create your future. Whatever you dream is possible. The universe wants you to fulfill your dreams and achieve all your desires. The difficult part is getting clear about what you want and then having the faith and perseverance to make it happen. Allow yourself to put time and energy into understanding what you would like your life to look like and feel like. What accomplishments would you like to achieve? Where would you like to go? Who would you like to be with? The clearer your intention, the more you can build your future according to your hopes and dreams. What do you really want to get done in this lifetime? You are free to create whatever you want in this world.

exercise

Future-Building Exercise

What do you really want to get done in this lifetime? You are free to create whatever you want in this world. The more specific you are, the easier it is to plan. Your hopes and dreams must be thought about and planned for to make them happen.

You may want to do this in a journal. Consider this exercise a personal trainer for your muscle that sees into and creates your future. You are not going to show this list to anyone, so just write without self-consciousness.

Write down all the things you need to get done or want to get done by:

1. the end of the day tomorrow _____

_____

_____

2. the end of the week _____

_____

_____

_____

3. the end of this month _____

_____

_____

_____

4. the end of next month _____

_____

_____

_____

5. New Year's Day

a. what's the year?_____

b. how old will you be?_____

c. how old will your loved ones be?_____

d. what are all the things you want to have done by that time?_____

_____

_____

_____

_____

_____

_____

_____

_____

6. New Year's Day, two years from now. Again write down the following:

a. what's the year?_____

b. how old will you be?_____

c. how old will your loved ones be?_____

d. what are all the things you want to have done by that time?_____

_____

_____

_____

_____

_____

_____

_____

7. New Year's Day, five years from now. Again write down the following:

a. what's the year?_____

b. how old will you be?_____

c. how old will your loved ones be?_____

d. what are all the things you want to have done by that time?_____

_____

_____

_____

_____

_____

_____

_____

8. in 10 years_____

_____

_____

_____

_____

_____

_____

9. in 20 years_____

_____

_____

_____

_____

_____

_____

Now remember this is your life. Make it happen!

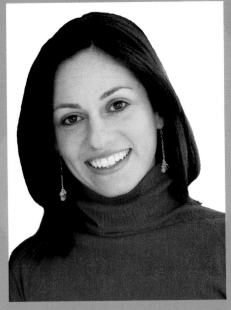

i started having terrible digestive problems when I was 13. At 18, I was diagnosed with Crohn's disease, and for the next seven years I tried every drug out there to get some relief from this major digestive disorder. As a last resort, I turned to nutrition my senior year of college, and improved my health significantly by eating higher quality foods. After graduation I really wanted to work with people who were like me, people who had health problems and wanted to get well. That's when a friend introduced me to Integrative Nutrition.

For so long I had been searching for that one perfect thing that would solve all my health problems, along with everyone else's. What I enjoyed about Integrative Nutrition was realizing that there is no one right approach to health, that there are many theories that work for different reasons, and the reason they work or don't work is based on the individual. I had never understood why things that helped other people with Crohn's weren't helping me. Integrative Nutrition showed me that health and healing is not one-size-fits-all. Learning how to care for my own unique body was a real lesson in self-discovery.

The other incredible aspect of Integrative Nutrition was the business training. The detailed information they gave us about how to start a business, along with all the tools we could possibly need, was the foundation for my career as a health counselor. When I came to school I was 23, and I've been in business for five years. The fact that I was confident enough at such a young age to get out there and start doing this work—and that I am still doing it today—speaks volumes to what they teach.

Debbie Sarfati
Graduate 2001
Boulder, CO
www.wholenourishment.com

My practice is in Boulder, Colorado, and it's really, really successful. I work with my private clients three days a week, and two days a week I work at a fitness center with their members. I also teach cooking classes twice a month. Recently, I wrote a nutrition and lifestyle program that is going to be sold with a fitness product in the U.S. and 18 different countries. I absolutely love health counseling. It's such a dynamic field and there are so many opportunities. I couldn't imagine doing anything else.

recipes

Let food be thy medicine
and medicine be thy food

Hippocrates

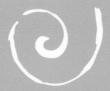

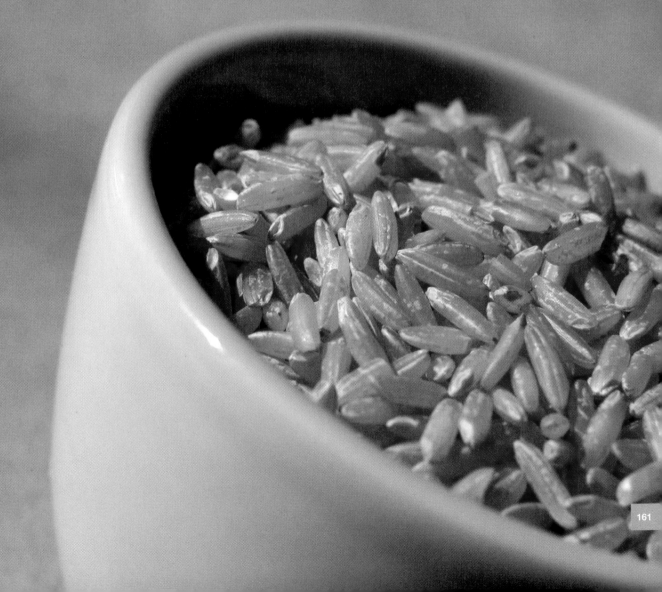

top 10 secrets to cooking the best grains

1. Use organic, unrefined whole grains. Quality matters.
2. Store your grains in an airtight container.

Before cooking:

3. Gently wash your grains in cold water. This reawakens dormant energy.
4. Soak them anywhere between 1 and 12 hours. This will eliminate phytic acid and help with digestion.
5. Dry-toast grains in a skillet over medium heat until they smell nutty. This enhances their natural flavor, allows them to cook more evenly, and decreases bitterness.

During cooking:

6. Use a pinch of sea salt or add pieces of sea vegetables. This adds flavor and nutritional enhancement.
7. A splash of olive oil helps prevent grains from sticking together.
8. Do not stir, as this makes them mushy and they lose water.
9. When grains hit boiling point, reduce heat to low, cover and let simmer for the suggested time.

After cooking:

10. Mix grains in the pot, allowing them to gently steam; cover for 10 minutes.

The 11th secret: Your energy as a cook is just as important as the quality of the food that you are using. Keep your energy positive and joyful around food. What you put into the food will come back when you eat it.

Morning Glory with Oats

2 cups rolled oats
4 cups water
$^1/_2$ cup raisins
$^1/_4$ cup almonds
$^1/_4$ cup sunflower seeds
$^1/_2$ teaspoon cinnamon
1 grated apple
Grated orange peel

Combine all ingredients except the apple and orange peel in a pot.
Bring to boil. Reduce heat to low.
Add apple and orange peel.
Continue cooking until water is absorbed and oats become nice and creamy. It will take 15 minutes total.
TIP: Add 1 heaping tablespoon raw honey or maple syrup.
TIP: You can also add more cinnamon or 1 teaspoon vanilla extract.

Muesli

1 cup rolled oats
2 cups almond or soy milk
5 to 6 cups dates
$^1/_2$ cup sunflower seeds

Soak all ingredients overnight covered, and it will be done by the morning. Without cooking!
TIP: Add shredded coconut, raisins or a tablespoon of brown rice syrup before eating.

Basic Brown Rice

1 cup brown rice
2 cups water
Pinch of sea salt

Presoak rice. Gently rinse rice.
Add water and salt. Bring to boil.
Cover. Reduce heat to low.
Simmer for 50 minutes if it is short grain, and 35 minutes if it is long grain basmati rice.
When it is done, pull from heat and let stand covered for 10 more minutes.
Fluff rice with fork before serving.

Golden Rice

2 cups white basmati rice

4 cups water

$^1/_2$ teaspoon turmeric

$^1/_2$ teaspoon cumin seeds

$^1/_4$ teaspoon sea salt

Wash and drain rice.

Add water and spices.

Mix gently before putting over heat.

Bring to boil, reduce heat and cover.

Simmer for 35 minutes.

When finished, remove from heat and tenderly fold rice. In this dish, spices tend to dry out rice, so add 1 teaspoon ghee or 1 tablespoon olive oil if needed.

Sesame Dulse Brown Rice

2 cups brown rice

4 cups water

$^1/_2$ cup toasted black sesame seeds

$^1/_4$ cup dulse

Wash and drain rice.

Add water and put over medium-high heat.

Meanwhile, toast sesame seeds in a skillet over medium heat.

Seeds are done when they release their full, nutty flavor into the air.

Add dulse to seeds. You may have to tear dulse into small pieces before adding it.

When water reaches a boil, add the seeds and dulse.

Mix, cover and simmer for 45 minutes.

TIP: *More information about sea vegetables like dulse, hiziki, arame, kombu and nori is given later in this chapter.*

Wild Rice

1 cup wild rice

4 cups water

Pinch of sea salt

Wash and drain rice.

Bring rice and water to a boil.

Add salt.

Turn heat to low, cover and simmer for 45 to 50 minutes.

Your grain is ready when black seeds are opened up.

Mix and serve.

Very Easy Fried Rice

1 tablespoon olive oil

1 small onion

2 cloves shredded garlic

1 medium diced carrot

1/2 bunch scallion

Grated ginger

4 cups cooked long grain brown rice

2 tablespoons tamari soy sauce

1 teaspoon toasted sesame oil

Sauté onion in olive oil.

Shred garlic into onion.

Add carrot and sauté for 4 minutes.

Add scallion. Add ginger.

Sauté these for about 4 more minutes so flavors can melt into each other.

Add rice and sprinkle with water. Water gives extra steam to the dish.

Add tamari soy sauce and toasted sesame oil.

Lower heat and cook for 10 more minutes, stirring occasionally.

TIP: Garnish with chopped parsley before serving.

Gypsies' Singing Rice Salad

1 cup cooked brown basmati rice

1 cup cooked white basmati rice

1 red bell pepper

1 medium purple onion

2 stalks celery

1 cup parsley

1/2 cup white sesame seeds

1/2 cup pumpkin seeds

2 tablespoons olive oil

1/4 teaspoon black pepper

If you use leftover rice, put it in the steaming basket to re-energize it and steam for 10 minutes.

Otherwise, cook according to basic rice preparation method.

Chop bell pepper and onion.

Dice celery.

Chop parsley.

Toast sesame and pumpkin seeds. You can combine them when you toast them. Make sure you don't let them get dark brown.

Combine all ingredients in a big bowl, adding olive oil and black pepper.

TIP: Add zest to it by squeezing 1/2 a lemon and adding 1/3 cup chopped mint leaves.

Buckwheat with Carrot and Arame

$^1/_2$ cup arame

1 large carrot

1 cup raw buckwheat

1$^2/_3$ cups water

Soak arame.

Shred carrot.

Dry-toast grains until nutty and golden brown.

Bring water to boil.

Slowly add buckwheat, bring back to a boil, reduce heat and cover. Simmer for 15 minutes.

Remove from heat and let sit for 5 minutes.

Rinse arame and mix with shredded carrot to buckwheat.

TIP: Add toasted sesame oil and sprinkle with fresh scallion.

Very Russian Buckwheat

1 cup buckwheat

1 cup water

1 cup sauerkraut juice

$^1/_2$ cup sauerkraut

Dry-toast grains.

Mix water with the sauerkraut juice and bring to boil.

Add grains slowly, reduce heat, then cover. Simmer for 15 minutes.

Remove from heat and keep covered for 5 minutes.

Add sauerkraut, mix and serve.

TIP: You can add sautéed onions, minced scallion, garlic, pepper or even scrambled eggs.

Millet with Roasted Sunflower Seeds

1 cup millet

$^1/_2$ cup sunflower seeds

3 cups water

Pinch of sea salt

Wash and drain millet.

Dry-toast sunflower seeds in a skillet over medium heat until they smell nutty, approximately 4 minutes.

Bring water to boil.

Add millet and seeds.

Cover and simmer for 30 minutes.

When done, fluff and let sit for 10 minutes. Mix, serve and devour.

TIP: If millet is too dry for you, add more water when cooking. Or add a tablespoon of olive oil when it is done.

TIP: To dress up any millet dish, use scallion, parsley, cilantro or sautéed onion.

Millet–Carrot–Hiziki–Burdock

2 stalks scallion

2 tablespoons olive oil, divided

2 shredded carrots

3-inch piece thinly sliced burdock root

1 cup millet

$\frac{1}{4}$-inch piece soaked, rinsed hiziki

6 cups water

Gomasio to garnish

Sauté scallion in 1 tablespoon of olive oil. Add carrots and sauté for 4 minutes.

Add sliced burdock, millet. and hiziki.

Let these aromas get friendly with each other by sautéing them over medium heat for about 3 more minutes.

Add water and bring to a boil. Cover and cook over low heat for 30 minutes.

When it is done, the millet and hiziki will be moist and full of aroma.

Mix and let sit covered for 5 minutes.

Add remaining olive oil, sprinkle with gomasio, and serve.

Winter Squash and Millet

1 small chopped onion

1 small peeled and cubed acorn squash

3 cups millet

8-inch piece kombu

$7\frac{1}{2}$ cups water

1 tablespoon olive oil

Sauté onion until it is golden brown.

Add squash; sauté them together for 3 minutes.

Add millet and kombu.

Add water, bring to boil, then reduce heat and cover. Cook for 30 minutes or until water is evaporated.

Remove from heat, let stand for a few minutes. Fluff with fork, add olive oil and serve.

Spring Out Quinoa

2 cups quinoa

$3\frac{1}{2}$ cups water

1 bag peppermint tea

1 tablespoon olive oil

Fresh mint, basil and cilantro

Wash grains. Place them in water and add peppermint tea bag.

Bring to a boil. Cover and simmer for 15 to 20 minutes, then remove from heat and let stand for 5 minutes.

When it is done, add olive oil and fluff.

Garnish with chopped fresh herbs and serve.

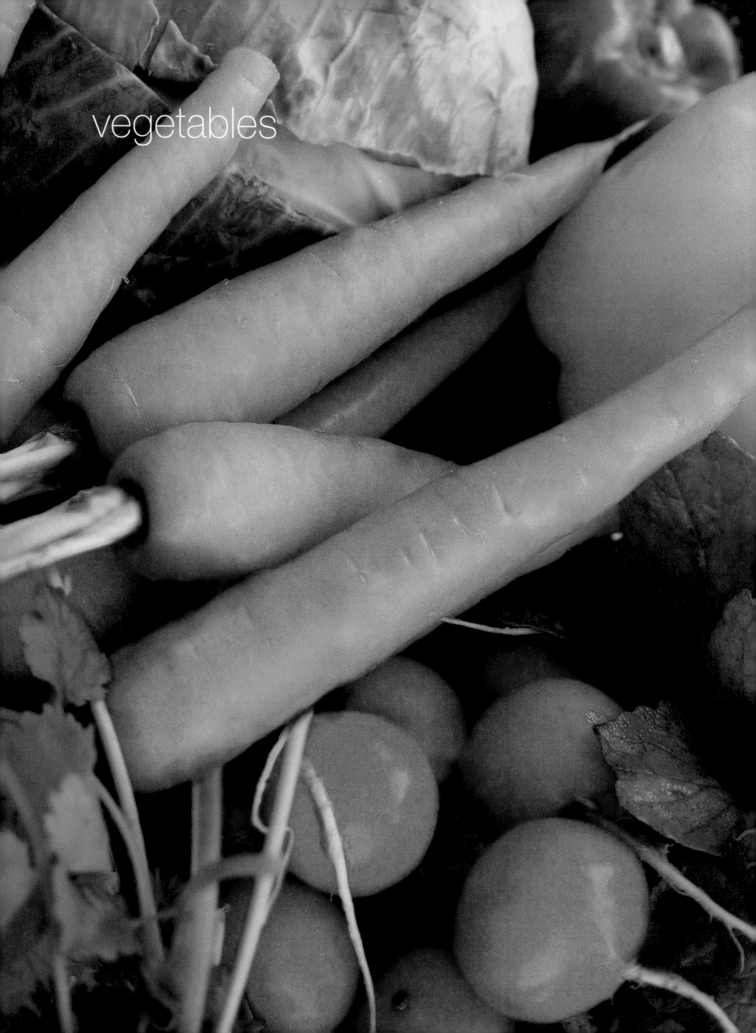

vegetables

basic cooking methods for vegetables

Steaming Steaming is a simple way to cook vegetables, allowing you to experience their simple flavors in a pure form. Steaming takes 5 to10 minutes for leafy green vegetables, and 10 to 25 minutes for root vegetables. All you need is a steaming basket, a pot with about 2 inches of water at the bottom, and a lid. This is a great cooking option in the summer months when a large range of farm-fresh vegetables, with all their beautiful colors, are available.

Stir-Frying Stir-frying is another quick and nutritious way to prepare vegetables. This method highlights vegetables' natural flavors. It takes just 5 to 10 minutes. You can stir-fry in oil or water. The softer the vegetables are, the less time they take to cook. All you need is a skillet with a lid. If you choose to use oil, heat a skillet and add 3 to 5 tablespoons of the oil. Add vegetables and sprinkle them with a pinch of sea salt to enhance their flavor. You can stir-fry garlic, ginger or dried herbs of your choice in olive oil before adding veggies to give your dish a full body and exciting flavor. To reduce the amount of fat but keep the flavor, you can use 2 to 3 tablespoons of water and 1 tablespoon of oil. This is called a wet sauté. After stir-frying the veggies for a few minutes in the oil, add the water and cover to give the vegetables extra steam and heat. Another option is a pure water sauté. Place 1 inch of water in your skillet and add garlic, ginger or spices if desired. Bring to boil, add thinly sliced vegetables, cover and simmer for 5 to 10 minutes.

Baking Certain vegetables taste best baked. Baking brings out the very essence of the vegetables, especially squashes and roots. You need a baking pan or sheet, vegetables, an oven heated between 375 and 450 degrees, and 50 to 60 minutes of cooking time. Be sure to use a nonstick pan or oil the vegetables so they don't stick. This is a great option for those cooler months. The heat of the roasted vegetables can help keep you warm.

Quick Boiling When quick boiling vegetables, put them in boiling water and leave for 3 to 5 minutes. This method removes their raw flavor, makes them more digestible and brightens their color. When you're done boiling, rinse vegetables with cold water to stop additional cooking and to preserve the color. You can save the boiled water, which has been flavored and nutritionally enhanced through the cooking process, and use it for drinking, cooking grains, watering your plants or adding to soups.

vegetables to try

Leafy Green Vegetables
Collard greens

Kale – dinosaur kale, purple
    kale, lucinato kale

Dandelion greens

Mustard greens

Chard – Swiss chard, red
    chard, rainbow chard

Beet greens

Watercress

Parsley

Bok choy

Lettuces

Roots and Squashes
Carrot

Parsnip

Turnip

Rutabaga

Celery root

Burdock root

Acorn squash

Kabocha squash

Butternut squash

Delicata squash

The Fat Burners
Daikon radish

Leek

Scallion

Turnip

Onion

Celery

Shitaki mushrooms

Cabbage Family
Broccoli

Cauliflower

All cabbages

Brussels sprout

how to make plain, steamed vegetables more exciting

These hints can be applied to all steamed vegetables:

• After cooking, add 1 tablespoon olive oil or toasted sesame oil to every
2 cups of greens.

• Add 2 bay leaves or 1 teaspoon cumin seeds to the cooking water.

• Sprinkle cooked greens with toasted pumpkin, sesame, flax or sunflower seeds.
Or sprinkle with almonds, walnuts or dried shredded coconut.

• Sprinkle greens with fresh herbs: mint, dill, basil, parsley, cilantro, scallion.

• Use tamari soy sauce or umeboshi vinegar to add extra flavor to cooked veggies.

• Squeeze fresh lemon or lime juice over steamed vegetables.

• After steaming, quickly stir-fry with a pinch of sea salt, olive oil and garlic.

Steamed Kale

1 bunch of kale

Wash and cut kale.

Cut leaves into long strips or little, bite-size pieces.

The stems of kale can also be used. If desired, chop the stems.

Put about 2 inches of water in your pot.

Place basket into pot.

Place kale in steaming basket. If using stems, put these on the bottom.

Bring to boil, cover, lower heat and let steam for 5 minutes.

TIP: *Try this same technique with collard greens, bok choy and mustard greens.*

Sautéed Greens in Olive Oil

½ bunch mustard greens

½ bunch kale

½ bunch dandelion greens

1 tablespoon olive oil

2 cloves minced garlic

Fresh lemon juice or umeboshi vinegar to taste

Wash and chop greens.

Heat olive oil.

Add garlic and sauté for a few seconds.

Add greens and stir until all leaves are wilted, about 5 minutes.

Sprinkle with lemon juice or umeboshi vinegar.

Garlic Steamed String Beans

1 pound string beans

2 cloves shredded garlic

2 tablespoons tamari soy sauce

4 tablespoons tahini

Juice of ½ lemon

Wash and cut beans, taking care to chop ends off.

Place beans in a steaming basket.

Add about 2 inches of water to your pot.

Bring to boil, cover and steam for 10 minutes.

Meanwhile, mix garlic, tamari and tahini.

When beans are done, put them in serving bowl and pour garlic mixture over it.

Squeeze lemon on top and serve.

Bok Choy Stir-Fry

1 bunch bok choy

1/2 red bell pepper

2 cloves minced garlic

2 tablespoons olive oil

Pinch of sea salt

Wash bok choy and separate greens from stems.

Dice red pepper and garlic.

Heat oil.

Add garlic and sauté for a few seconds.

Add peppers and salt.

Make sure you stir to keep garlic from burning.

Add bok choy stems first and cook for a few minutes.

Next add the greens and stir until they become wilted.

TIP: You can add tamari soy sauce or fresh ginger juice to this dish.

Garlic Gingered Broccoli with Toasted Pumpkin Seeds

1 bunch broccoli

3 cloves garlic

5-inch piece fresh ginger

6 cups water

1 tablespoon olive oil

2 tablespoons tamari soy sauce

Wash and cut broccoli into florets.

You can use the stems, but it will take longer to cook.

Mince garlic.

Finely grate ginger.

Add 6 cups water to a pot.

Bring to boil.

Drop your broccoli in, and let quick boil for about 3 minutes.

Remove from water and give them a quick rinse.

Heat skillet with oil, add garlic and sauté for a few seconds before adding broccoli. Sauté them together, add tamari soy sauce and ginger juice.

TIP: Try this dish with cauliflower or brussels sprouts.

TIP: Garnish with finely chopped fresh tarragon or basil before serving.

Steamed Daikon Radish with Black Sesame Seeds

¹/₄ cup black sesame seeds

2 large daikon radishes

1 tablespoon olive oil

1 tablespoon umeboshi vinegar

Toast sesame seeds by placing them on a heated skillet.

Stir until they smell nutty. Remove from heat and set aside.

Wash radishes. If you have a stiff little brush that you can use for this purpose, then you don't have to worry about peeling; just scrub them well under running water.

Cut radishes in half-moon shapes, lengthwise first, then across.

Put them into steaming basket, bring 1 to 2 inches of water at bottom of pot to boil, cover and steam for 3 minutes.

When radishes are done, sprinkle them with the toasted sesame seeds, olive oil and umeboshi vinegar.

Sautéed Cabbage

2 cups cabbage

1 green apple

1 medium onion

2 tablespoons olive oil

2 tablespoons umeboshi vinegar

1 teaspoon mustard seeds

1 teaspoon caraway seeds

Finely slice the cabbage, apple and onion separately.

Heat oil in skillet.

Add and sauté onion.

Add umeboshi vinegar, mustard seeds and caraway seeds.

Sauté them together for 2 minutes.

Add cabbage and sauté for another 2 minutes.

Add apple.

Cover and simmer on low heat until cabbage is wilted and soft, approximately 10 minutes.

TIP: Garnish with gomasio or toasted pumpkin seeds.

Beet–Carrot–Parsnip–Fennel Extravaganza

5 small beets

3 big carrots

2 parsnips

1 fennel bulb

2 tablespoons olive oil

1/2 teaspoon sea salt

Preheat oven to 425 degrees.

Scrub all your vegetables.

Chop vegetables into 2-inch pieces and fennel bulb finely.

Mix vegetables with oil and sea salt. Transfer them to a baking dish.

Bake covered for 30 minutes. Uncover and bake for 15 minutes.

Roasted Rutabaga with Celery Root

1 rutabaga

1 celery root

2 tablespoons olive oil

1/2 teaspoon sea salt

1 teaspoon fresh rosemary

Preheat oven to 400 degrees.

Wash and scrub vegetables. Cut them into 1-inch-thick rounds.

Mix with oil, salt and rosemary.

Cover and bake for 30 minutes. Turn vegetables over and bake uncovered for 10 more minutes.

Collards with Dill and Parsley

1 bunch collard greens

2 tablespoons olive oil

1 teaspoon black pepper

Pinch of sea salt

1 cup chopped fresh dill

1 cup chopped fresh parsley

Wash collards, cut stems off, chop stems into small pieces and put aside. Stack leaves and roll them up, as you would a sushi roll, then slice from the end to create long strips.

Warm oil in a pan with black pepper and add stems, sautéing for a few minutes.

Add collard leaves and sea salt, then sauté for about 3 minutes.

Add water, cover and allow to steam for about 3 to 4 minutes, then remove from heat.

Add chopped dill and parsley, toss well and allow to sit uncovered for a few minutes, then serve.

TIP: Mix the juice of a lime and a dash of cayenne. Toss with the greens for a little extra kick!

Carrot Burdock Power Meal

1 onion
1 large burdock root
1 large carrot
1 teaspoon olive oil
Pinch of sea salt

Wash and chop vegetables into odd shapes.
Heat oil in skillet.
Sauté veggies together with a pinch of sea salt over medium-high heat about 5 minutes.
Add ¹/₂ inch of water to skillet, cover and simmer for 10 to 15 minutes on low heat.
TIP: Try serving with a sprinkle of toasted seeds or fresh parsley for variety.

Baked Caraway Sweet Potato with Rosemary

3 medium sweet potatoes
2 tablespoons olive oil
4¹/₂ cups fresh rosemary
¹/₂ tablespoon caraway seeds

Preheat oven to 400 degrees.
Scrub sweet potatoes under running water and cut them into big chunks.
Sprinkle baking dish with oil, place the sweet potatoes into the dish, and add rosemary and caraway seeds.
Mix all ingredients together.
Cover and bake for 50 minutes.
TIP: Rosemary and caraway seeds can be substituted with cinnamon and 2 tablespoons of maple syrup.

Veggie Bake

All the leftover veggies in your fridge that need to be used up
1 large can chopped tomatoes
1 can chickpeas
3 or 4 large yams, thinly sliced
Extra virgin olive oil

Preheat oven to 160 degrees.
Chop veggies (not yams) and stir-fry in a bit of oil until soft.
Add can of tomatoes and drained can of chickpeas.
In a casserole or lasagna dish, layer yams then veggie mix (same as if you were making lasagna,
but use potatoes as lasagna sheets and veggie mix instead of meat).
Finish with a layer of yams, lightly drizzle olive oil on top.
Bake for 30 minutes. Then take off cover, turn up temperature to 180 degrees for 10 minutes to crisp
up the top later.
TIP: Add your favorite spices, like basil, oregano, fennel, cumin, chilli pepper, sea salt, etc. when adding tomatoes and chickpeas.

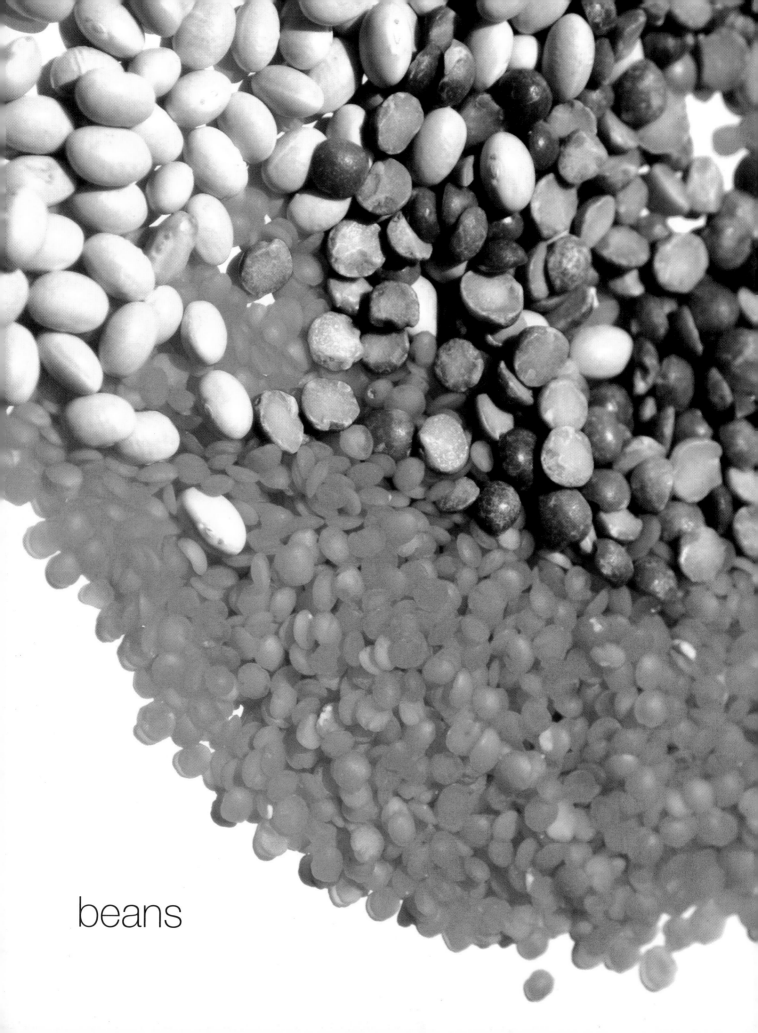

beans

soaking beans

If you are new to beans, introduce them slowly, allowing your digestive system time to adjust and learn how to break them down. Soaking will make beans more digestible by reducing complex sugars.

There are two options for soaking:

Quick Soak – Boil the beans in water for 5 minutes, remove from heat, cover and allow them to soak for 2 to 4 hours (soaking longer does not damage). Drain, rinse, add to fresh water and proceed with cooking.

Overnight Soak – Soak beans 8 to 12 hours, drain, rinse, add to fresh water and proceed with cooking.

A simple way to tell if you have soaked your beans enough is to slice a bean in half; if the center is still opaque, soak more.

basic bean cooking guide

- Wash and clean beans.

- Soak beans using either of the two methods above.

- Do not cook beans in water they were soaked in.

- Place beans in heavy pot with suggested amount of water.

- Bring to boil.

- Skim off the foam.

- Cook beans with a 1- to 3-inch strip of kombu (a sea vegetable), which makes them more digestible and adds flavor and minerals.

- Spices that aid digestion are bay leaf, cumin, anise and fennel. These can be added to the water while cooking.

- Cover, reduce heat and simmer for the suggested time.

- Only add salt towards the end of cooking, approximately 10 minutes before beans are done. Otherwise, it will interfere with thorough cooking.

pressure cooking guide for beans

- Wash and clean beans.

- Soak beans using either of the two methods above.

- Add beans to pressure cooker.

- Also add soaked 1- to 3-inch strip of kombu with beans.

- Cover and bring to pressure.

- Reduce heat and cook for the suggested time.

- Remove cover, season and cook uncovered until water evaporates.

Bean Cooking Time Chart	
BEAN VARIETY	MINIMUM COOKING TIME
Aduki beans	$1^1/_2$ hours
Black beans	45 to 60 minutes
Chickpeas	$1^1/_2$ hours
Kidney beans	$1^1/_2$ hours
Brown lentils	45 minutes
French lentils	30 to 45 minutes
Red lentils	20 to 25 minutes
Pinto beans	1 hour
Split peas	1 hour

canned beans

A busy lifestyle does not always allow time for soaking and cooking dried beans. Having canned beans on hand provides a quick meal option. Some people even find that canned beans are easier to digest than dried, soaked beans. When buying canned beans, there are a few things to consider:

- Buy canned beans that do not contain added salt or preservatives.

- Look for beans that have been cooked with kombu, which aids digestion.

- Some companies, such as Eden and Westbrae, line their cans so the beans are not sitting in tin. This is preferable.

- Rinse beans once removed from the can.

Basic Aduki Beans

1 cup aduki beans

5-inch piece kombu

4 cups water

2 bay leaves

1 teaspoon sea salt

Wash beans.

Soak kombu until it starts to soften, about 10 minutes.

Place kombu and aduki beans in a pot.

Cover with water.

Bring to a boil.

Add bay leaves.

Cover and simmer for 1 hour.

Allow beans to cook until they are soft enough for your taste. Add salt.

TIP: To check for softness, take a couple of beans out from your pot and squeeze them between your thumb and pointer finger. If beans press easily, they are finished. If they feel hard in the middle, they need more time.

Aduki Squash Stew

1 small acorn squash

1$\frac{1}{2}$ cups aduki beans

3-inch piece kombu

3-inch piece wakame

5 cups water

2 tablespoons tamari soy sauce

Peel and cube squash into 2-inch squares.

Place washed beans and seaweed in pot with water.

Bring to boil.

Cover and simmer for 30 minutes.

Uncover and add squash cubes.

Cover and simmer for 30 more minutes.

Uncover, add tamari soy sauce and stir until water evaporates.

TIP: Try the same recipe with roots like carrot, parsnip and turnip. These roots require 10 minutes less cooking time with beans.

Red Lentil Burgers

2 cups red lentils
$1/4$ cup hiziki (optional)
1 medium chopped onion
2 cloves minced garlic
$1/2$ cup chopped fresh cilantro
3 cups water
$1/4$ tablespoon dried basil
$1/4$ tablespoon dried cumin
$1/8$ tablespoon turmeric
$1/8$ tablespoon thyme
2 tablespoons tamari soy sauce
1 tablespoon umeboshi vinegar

Wash and drain lentils and hiziki.

In a pot, sauté onion, garlic and cilantro.

Add lentils and hiziki.

Add water and bring to a boil.

Add spices, tamari and umeboshi vinegar, cover and simmer for 10 minutes.

Uncover, stir and cover again for another 10 minutes.

Stir and simmer vigorously uncovered for 3 more minutes.

It will look mushy because red lentils lose their shape when cooking.

Place lentils in a bowl and into the fridge to cool. When cool, form burgers 4 inches in diameter.

Sprinkle with chopped scallion and serve with brown rice and greens.

TIP: You can toast burgers in a toaster oven or broiler to give them a crispy golden brown outside.

Basic Chickpeas

1 cup chickpeas
2 cups water
5-inch piece kombu
Pinch of sea salt

Wash beans.

Place them in pressure cooker with water and kombu. Cover.

Bring to pressure.

Reduce heat and cook for 1 hour.

TIP: You can make delicious salads by adding chopped vegetables, sea vegetables (hiziki, arame), onions, scallion, dill, basil and other herbs.

Hummus

2 cups cooked chickpeas

1/3 cup chickpea water left over from pressure cooker

3 tablespoons tahini

3 cloves garlic

1/2 teaspoon sea salt

2 tablespoons fresh lemon juice

1/4 teaspoon black pepper

1/8 teaspoon cumin

1/8 teaspoon coriander

Blend all ingredients until smooth. Serve with pita bread or chopped raw veggies.

TIP: Use canned beans to save time.

TIP: For richer flavor, sauté onions and garlic and add to blender.

TIP: Garnish with dill, scallion or cilantro.

Vegetarian Bean Chili

1 tablespoon olive oil

1 chopped onion

2 to 3 cloves minced garlic

1 carrot, cut into quarter moons

1 chopped red, green or yellow pepper

1 teaspoon each chili powder, ground cumin, dried oregano

3 cups cooked or canned red, black or kidney beans

1 cup water or vegetable stock

2 tablespoons umeboshi vinegar or organic tomato paste

1 teaspoon sea salt

Heat oil in a large heavy pan.

Add onions and garlic and sauté until the onions start to brown.

Add the rest of the vegetables, chili powder, cumin and oregano.

Sauté for 5 minutes.

Add the rest of the ingredients.

Cover and simmer for 10 to15 minutes.

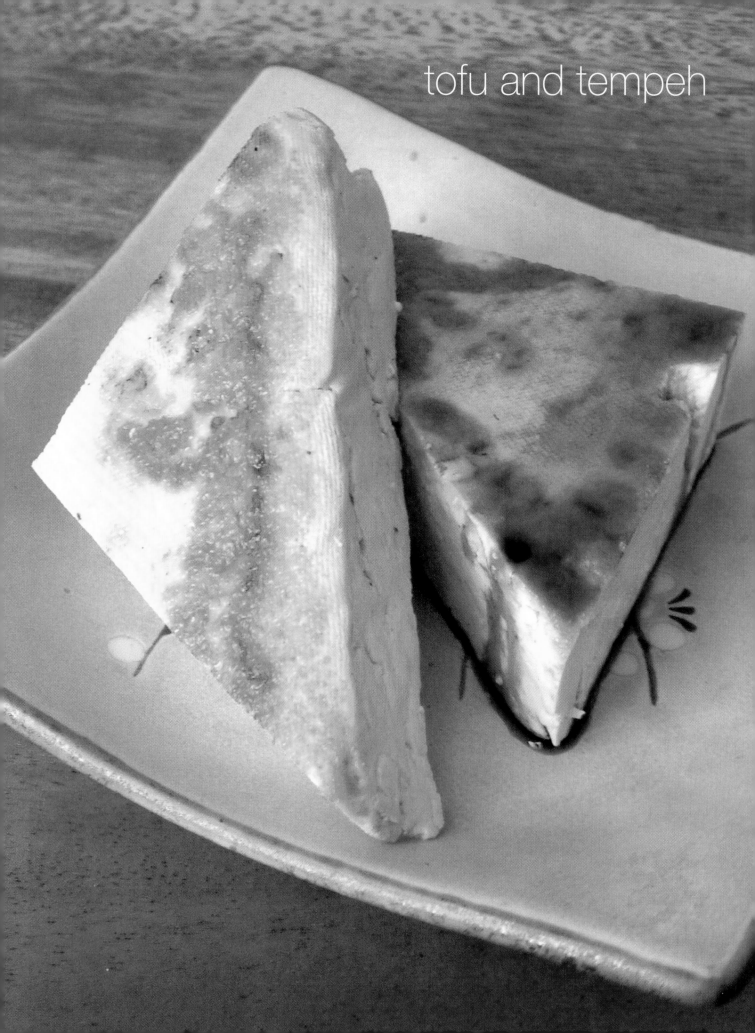

tofu and tempeh

Tofu and Tempeh

Tofu and tempeh are made from the soybean. Soy and tofu products are a versatile vegetarian protein option. If you are enthusiastic about tofu and enjoy experimenting, you can use it to create savory dips, mayonnaise, whipped cream and a variety of desserts. Recipes for tofu dishes are available in many vegetarian cookbooks. Here are some basic tofu and tempeh dishes.

Marinated Tofu Stir-Fry

1 block firm tofu
2 to 3 tablespoons olive oil
2 tablespoons sesame oil

Marinade:
1 tablespoon ginger juice
$1/2$ tablespoon tamari soy sauce
$1/2$ cup brown rice vinegar
$1/2$ cup toasted sesame oil
$1/2$ cup chopped fresh cilantro
2 cloves shredded garlic

Drain liquid from tofu.
Press excess water from tofu by placing it in a strainer over a bowl. Cover tofu with plate and place a heavy object on top, pressing the tofu. Leave for 1 hour.
Cut tofu into 1-inch squares after draining.
Set tofu aside and prepare marinade by mixing all ingredients.
Marinate tofu for 30 minutes or overnight.
Heat olive oil and sesame oil in skillet.
Add tofu and quick stir-fry until tofu becomes golden brown.

Scrambled Tofu

1 block firm tofu

2 to 3 tablespoons olive oil

$1/2$ teaspoon tamari soy sauce

$1/8$ teaspoon turmeric

1 red onion

$1/2$ red bell pepper

$1/8$ teaspoon paprika

1 tablespoon umeboshi vinegar

Dash of black pepper

Press tofu as described above to remove excess water and then crumble into small pieces.

Heat oil.

Add tofu, tamari and turmeric.

Sauté for a few minutes.

Chop onion and pepper.

Add vegetables, paprika, umeboshi vinegar and black pepper to tofu.

Cook for 5 minutes or until mixture thoroughly heats and flavors blend.

TIP: Use alfalfa sprouts or fresh parsley to garnish.

Marinated Baked Tofu

1 block firm tofu

Marinade:

1 small onion

3 cloves minced garlic

1 cup water

4 tablespoons olive oil

2 tablespoons brown rice vinegar

1 tablespoon dried basil

1 tablespoon dried oregano

$1/2$ teaspoon black pepper

Dash of cayenne pepper or paprika

Rinse and press tofu.

Cut tofu into 1-inch square chunks.

Prepare marinade by mixing all ingredients.

Add tofu and marinate in the refrigerator for 1 hour.

Preheat oven to 375 degrees.

Place marinated tofu on baking sheet and bake until it is golden and crispy, about 10 to 15 minutes.

TIP: Garnish with parsley or sprouts.

Marinated Tempeh

8 ounces tempeh

1 tablespoon olive oil

Marinade:

1/2 cup water

1/2 tablespoon grated fresh ginger

1 tablespoon curry powder

1 tablespoon umeboshi vinegar or 1/2 teaspoon sea salt

1 teaspoon cumin

1 tablespoon brown rice vinegar or 1/2 cup fresh lemon juice

Mix ingredients for marinade.

Cut tempeh into strips.

Soak tempeh for 30 minutes in marinade.

Heat skillet, add oil and quickly stir-fry tempeh until it is golden brown.

Very Versatile Mashed Tempeh

1/2 cup soaked arame, hiziki or dulse

8 ounces tempeh

1 small red onion

1/2 bunch finely chopped scallion

2 tablespoons water

1/2 cup finely chopped celery or red bell pepper

1 tablespoon tahini

1 tablespoon ginger juice

1 tablespoon fresh lemon juice

Rinse, wash and soak sea vegetables for 20 minutes. (You don't have to soak dulse.)

Place tempeh, onion, scallion and sea vegetables in a pot with water and cook over low heat until they are soft and the water evaporates, about 30 minutes.

Transfer to a bigger bowl and mash with potato masher or fork.

Add celery or pepper, tahini, ginger juice and fresh lemon juice.

Mix very well.

TIP: Wrap this in whole sprouted grain wraps, whole wheat pita bread, nori or blanched, dark green vegetable leaves (collard greens or kale).

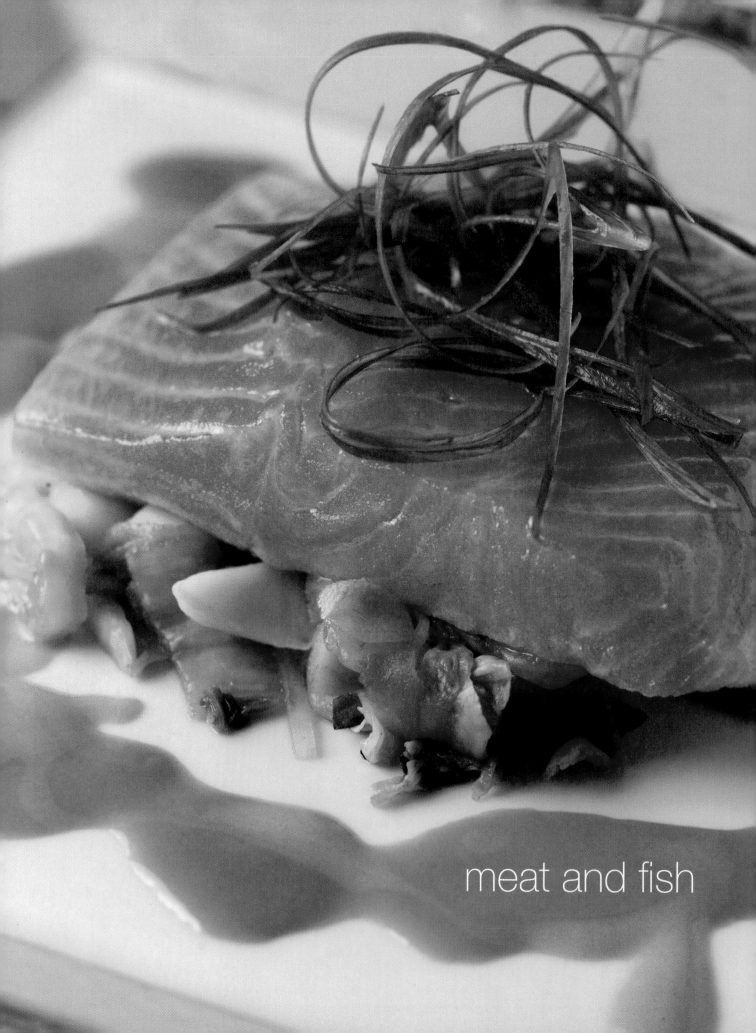

meat and fish

Salmon Cakes

4 ounces cooked salmon

6 rice crackers

1/2 onion

2 cloves minced garlic

1 tablespoon fresh lemon juice

Dash of black pepper

Dash of coriander

1 tablespoon olive oil

Break salmon and rice crackers into small pieces.

Mix all ingredients together.

Create several small patties.

Refrigerate for 1 hour.

In a skillet, heat oil on high.

Quickly fry both sides of each patty for 2 minutes.

TIP: *Serve with brown rice and lemon slices.*

Ideal Dill Fish

1 pound cod fish fillet

Dash of sea salt

Dash of black pepper

1/2 cup fresh dill

1 tablespoon fresh lemon juice

Rinse fish.

Season with salt and pepper.

Finely chop dill.

Fill skillet with about 1/2 inch of water and heat till steaming.

Drop in fish, cover top with dill and cook until it is soft, about 5 to 7 minutes.

Serve immediately.

Beef and Arugula Stir-Fry

$\frac{1}{2}$ pound sirloin, cut into 2- x $\frac{1}{8}$-inch strips

2 teaspoons olive oil

1 tablespoon minced fresh ginger

1 clove minced garlic

2 red bell peppers, cut into very thin strips

1 to 2 bunches well-washed arugula

2 teaspoons kuzu

2 tablespoons tamari

2 tablespoons brown rice or apple cider vinegar

$\frac{1}{4}$ cup water

Stir-fry the beef in a pan with 2 teaspoons of oil over medium-high heat for about 2 minutes, or until browned.

Remove beef with tongs or fork, allowing excess oil to drip off, and set side.

In same pan in remaining oil, stir-fry ginger and garlic for 2 to 3 minutes, and then add the bell pepper. Cook for another 2 to 3 minutes.

Mix together fresh arugula and bell pepper mixture in a serving bowl.

In a small bowl, combine kuzu, tamari, vinegar and water.

Place kuzu mixture into skillet and cook over medium heat until sauce starts to thicken.

Return the beef to the skillet and cook for 1 minute, just enough to warm up the beef.

Add the beef to the serving bowl with arugula and bell peppers.

Mix and serve warm.

Spicy Leek Meatballs

1 pound lean ground turkey or ground beef

1 tablespoon minced fresh ginger

2 minced fresh chili peppers

$1\frac{1}{2}$ cups minced leek (white and light green part only, about one bunch)

2 tablespoons flour (whole wheat, millet, rice, soy or whatever type you have on hand)

2 tablespoons sesame oil

Seasalt and pepper to taste

Place all the ingredients in a large mixing bowl.

Knead well by hand until the ingredients are thoroughly combined.

Divide the mixture into 10 to 12 equal portions, about $\frac{1}{4}$ cup each. Roll each portion into a ball.

Heat the cooking oil in a large nonstick pan over medium-high heat.

Add meatballs and pan-fry, covered, turning occasionally, until browned on all sides and cooked through, about 10 minutes.

Drain on paper towel.

TIP: Serve over a bed of simple steamed greens.

TIP: They freeze really well. A few can be taken out of the freezer and popped into a soup for a quick dinner option.

Chai Chicken

4 organic chicken legs

4 to 5 sliced carrots

1 cup coconut milk

2 cups chai tea

Chai is the Indian way of drinking tea. You can buy chai tea bags, or make it yourself by putting shredded ginger, cinnamon powder and ground cardamom seeds in a pot with 2 cups of water and bringing it to a boil. Cook for 2 to 3 minutes to bring flavor out of the spices, then add tea, stirring as you do so.

Preheat oven to 350 degrees.

Place sliced chicken and carrots in a casserole dish. Sprinkle with a pinch of salt and pepper.

In a pot, combine coconut milk and tea and bring to a boil.

Pour over the chicken in the casserole dish. Cover with lid and bake in the oven at 350 degrees for 45 minutes, or until chicken is cooked through.

Serve with brown basmati rice and greens. Use coconut milk mixture as a sauce.

Citrus Savory Chicken

$\frac{1}{2}$ cup fresh grapefruit juice (ruby red works best, but any kind will do)

1 tablespoon olive oil

1 tablespoon lime juice

2 cloves minced garlic

1 teaspoon dried basil

1 teaspoon dried rosemary

$\frac{1}{2}$ teaspoon sea salt

Pinch of cayenne

2 pinches red chili flakes

4 chicken breast halves on the bone

Combine the juice with all the ingredients and place in a zip-lock bag or bowl with chicken.

Allow to marinate in the fridge for at least 1hour, up to 3 hours.

Preheat oven to 375 degrees.

Place chicken with juice in a baking dish.

Bake covered for 20 minutes.

Uncover and bake for 25 more minutes or until chicken cooked through.

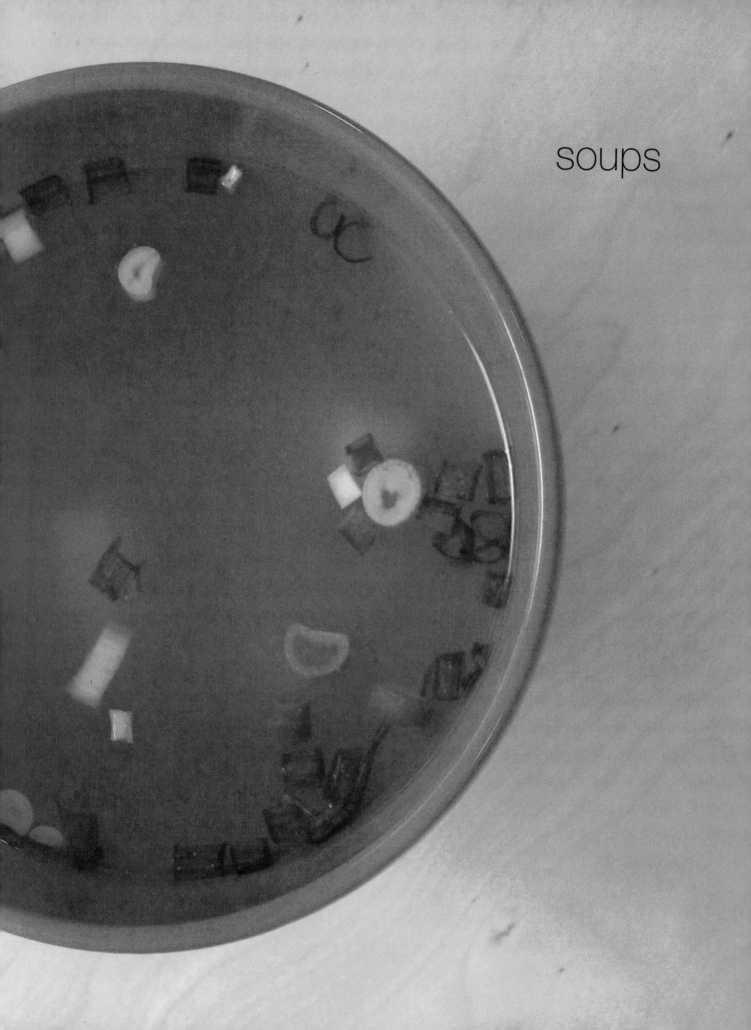

soups

Mighty Miso Soup

8-inch piece wakame

5-inch piece kombu

1 large onion

1 medium daikon radish

5 cups water

1 to 2 tablespoons barley miso

1 cup chopped scallion or leek

Wash and soak wakame and kombu for 3 minutes or until softened, and cut into little pieces.

Chop onion and daikon radish.

Add all vegetables and sea vegetables to water and bring to boil.

Do not add miso yet!

Reduce heat, cover and simmer soup broth for 10 minutes.

Meanwhile, remove 1 cup of liquid from the pot and dissolve miso paste in the liquid.

Return miso mixture to pot, reduce heat to very low and cook for 2 to 3 more minutes. Do not boil.

Garnish soup with scallion or leek.

Shiitake Miso Soup

8-inch piece kombu

8 dried shiitake mushrooms

1 cup fresh shiitake mushrooms

1 medium onion

1 large carrot

6 cups water

6 to 8 tablespoons barley miso

1 cup chopped fresh parsley

Soak kombu in water for 3 minutes or until softened, and cut into little pieces.

Soak dried mushrooms in water for 20 minutes. Remove stems and thinly slice fresh and dried mushrooms.

Dice onion and slice carrot into rounds.

Place water into a soup pot and bring to boil.

Add onion, carrot, shiitake mushrooms and kombu.

Do not add miso yet!

Reduce heat, cover and simmer soup broth for 10 minutes.

Meanwhile, remove 1 cup of liquid from the pot and dissolve miso paste in the liquid.

Return miso mixture to pot, reduce heat to very low and cook for 2 to 3 more minutes. Do not boil.

Garnish soup with parsley.

TIP: You can add other vegetables to your miso soup, including daikon radish, leek, snow peas, mustard greens and Chinese cabbage.

Easy Breezy Soup

Try any of these vegetable combinations to create a simply delicious soup:

Carrot, parsnip, celery, parsley.

Squash, carrot, ginger, beets.

Broccoli, onion, leek.

Daikon radish, leek, parsley, carrot.

Mustard greens, leek, onion.

Kale, cabbage, parsnip.

Use 5 cups water. Bring to boil.

Add 1 cup of each vegetable that you choose to cook.

Cover and simmer for 20 minutes.

TIP: Garnish with parsley and scallion. TIP: To add richness to soup, sauté 1 medium onion and add to water before cooking.

TIP: To make a pureed soup, place soup in a blender after cooking.

Carrot Ginger Soup

6 carrots

1 medium onion

1 teaspoon sea salt

4 cups water

6-inch piece fresh ginger

Fresh parsley to garnish

Wash, peel and cut carrots and onion into chunks.

Place vegetables and salt in a pot.

Add water. Bring to a boil. Cover with a lid.

Simmer on low heat for 25 minutes.

Transfer soup into blender, adding water if necessary to achieve desired consistency.

When blending is done, squeeze juice from grated ginger and add to soup. Garnish with parsley.

TIP: For extra flavor, sauté vegetables before cooking.

TIP: Substitute carrots with squash, parsnip or beets. Squash and beets need 35 to 40 minutes to cook.

Split Pea Soup

2 cups split peas

8 cups water

6-inch piece kombu

1 large chopped onion

2 large chopped carrots

2 chopped parsnips

½ cup chopped fresh dill

2 tablespoons tamari soy sauce

Soak peas for several hours. Wash peas.

Add water. Add kombu.

Bring to boil, skim off any foam.

Add onion.

Add more water if necessary and simmer over low heat for 30 minutes.

Add all other vegetables, dill and tamari and simmer, covered, for an additional 30 minutes.

Creamy Broccoli Soup

1 bunch broccoli

5 cups water

1 small onion

2 cloves garlic

2 tablespoons barley miso

1 cup cooked brown rice

Wash broccoli and separate stems from florets.

In a pot, bring water to a boil.

Add broccoli stems and onion.

Mince the garlic and add to the pot.

Reduce heat and simmer for 10 minutes.

Meanwhile, remove 2 cups of liquid from the pot, dissolve miso paste in the liquid, add brown rice, and return to the pot.

Put soup in the blender and blend. When it is smooth, return to the pot.

Add broccoli florets and cook 10 more minutes.

Chicken Ginger Soup

2$1/2$ pounds skinned chicken

3 long stocks celery

1 bunch scallion

3-inch piece fresh ginger, cut into slivers

Sea salt to taste

2 teaspoons fresh lemon juice

1 bunch chopped fresh parsley or cilantro

Place the chicken in a pot with enough water to cover it, then cover the pot and bring to a boil over medium-high heat.

Add celery, scallion and ginger.

Reduce heat and simmer, covered, for 1$1/2$ hours.

Remove the chicken, allow it to cool, then pull the meat from the bones.

Return chicken to the pot and add salt, lemon juice and parsley or cilantro.

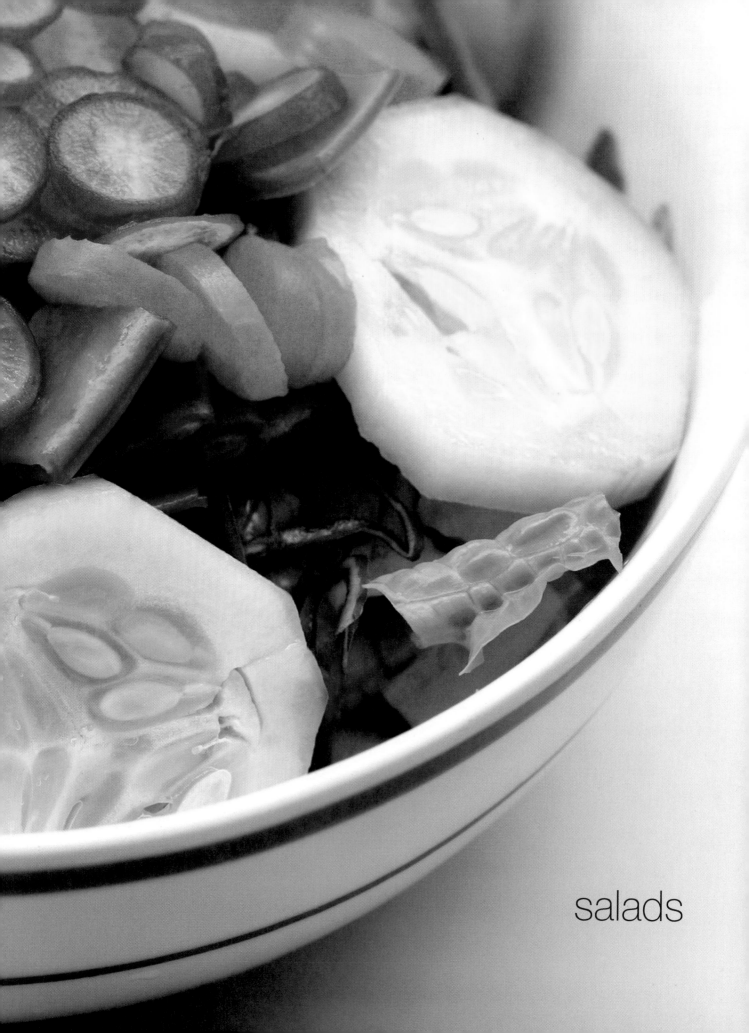

salads

Quinoa Salad

2 cups cooked quinoa

$1/2$ cup chopped radishes

$1/2$ cup chopped cucumber

$1/2$ cup chopped celery

$1/2$ cup chopped onion, preferably red

$1/2$ cup chopped fresh parsley

$1/2$ cup chopped red bell pepper

1 tablespoon olive oil

Combine all ingredients together in a big bowl.

Mix well.

TIP: *Garnish with cherry tomatoes and shredded garlic cloves and chill before serving.*

Black Bean Salad

2 cups black beans

5-inch piece kombu

4 cups water

$1/2$ onion

1 red and 1 yellow bell pepper

2 cloves garlic

1 teaspoon coriander

2 teaspoons cumin

Pinch of cayenne

1 teaspoon sea salt

1 tablespoon olive oil

Wash presoaked beans.

Place them in a pot with kombu.

Add water and bring to boil.

Cover and simmer for an hour.

Chop onion finely. Dice pepper. Mince garlic.

Sauté onions and garlic with spices and salt.

Mix cooked beans with sautéed onions and garlic in serving bowl.

Add peppers and olive oil.

TIP: *Garnish with cilantro and fresh lemon juice.*

2 cups French lentils

8-inch piece wakame or kombu

4 cups water

1 teaspoon dried thyme

1 teaspoon dried rosemary

2 medium chopped parsnips

8 to 10 dried shiitake mushrooms

2 tablespoons tamari soy sauce

4 cloves diced garlic

1 bunch chopped scallion

½ cup chopped fresh basil

2 tablespoons olive oil

½ teaspoon black pepper

½ cup dried, coarsely chopped chestnuts

Wash lentils.

Add lentils and wakame or kombu to water and bring to a boil.

Add thyme and rosemary.

Cover and simmer for 15 minutes over low heat.

Uncover and add chopped parsnip.

Cover and simmer for 15 more minutes.

Meanwhile, soak mushrooms for a few minutes and cut them into quarters.

Transfer lentils into a big bowl; add mushrooms, tamari, garlic, scallion, basil, olive oil and black pepper.

Add chestnuts.

TIP: You can add leftover or fresh grains of any kind.

2 cups green lentils

2 bay leaves

4 cups water

$1/4$ cup cumin

1 medium carrot

3 stalks celery

1 bunch scallion

1 bunch watercress

$1/2$ cup fresh mint

$1/4$ cup fresh basil

2 tablespoons olive oil

2 tablespoons tamari soy sauce

Pinch of sea salt

$1/2$ teaspoon black pepper

2 tablespoons fresh lemon juice

Wash and drain lentils.

Place them in a pot with bay leaves.

Add water and cumin.

Bring to a boil.

Cover and simmer for 30 to 45 minutes.

Check periodically for desired softness.

When soft, set aside, but leave covered.

Meanwhile, wash all vegetables.

Shred carrot. Chop celery, scallion and watercress.

Finely chop fresh mint and basil.

In a big bowl, mix chopped vegetables and lentils.

Add olive oil, tamari, salt, black pepper and lemon juice.

Pressed Salad

1 cucumber

1/2 cup onion

1/4 cup dulse

1 bunch scallion

1/2 leek

1 bunch red radishes

1 tablespoon brown rice vinegar

1 tablespoon umeboshi vinegar

Thinly slice cucumber and onion.

Rinse dulse and slice finely.

Chop scallion and only the green part of the leek. Thinly slice radishes.

Mix all ingredients except vinegar in a bowl.

Cover mixed salad, put a heavy object on top and let it press for 30 to 45 minutes.

When it is done, squeeze out excess water, add vinegar and it's ready to serve.

Cold Soba Noodle Salad

8 ounces soba noodles (100% buckwheat)

6 cups water

1 bunch chopped sprouted sunflower seeds or watercress

1/2 cup chopped red radishes

1/2 cup chopped celery

1/2 cup chopped cucumber

Put soba noodles into a pot of 6 cups boiling water.

Cook until tender, no more than 8 minutes.

Rinse with cold water when finished cooking.

Mix all vegetables and noodles.

Dressing:

1/2 cup finely chopped fresh basil

1 tablespoon toasted sesame oil

1/4 cup tahini

2 tablespoons tamari soy sauce

2-inch piece grated fresh ginger

Juice of 1/2 lemon

Mix all these ingredients and pour over noodles.

salad dressings

Element Dressing

1 cup toasted sesame seeds
1 cup water
1 tablespoon tamari soy sauce
1 tablespoon umeboshi vinegar
1 tablespoon brown rice syrup
1 tablespoon toasted sesame oil
1 tablespoon ginger juice

Mix in small bowl.

Tahini Lemon Dressing

2 tablespoons tahini
Juice of 1 lemon
$1/2$ cup water
$1/4$ tablespoon tamari soy sauce

Mix in small bowl.

Ginger Parsley Garlic Dressing

4-inch piece fresh ginger
1 bunch fresh parsley
2 cloves garlic
Juice of $1/2$ lemon
$1/2$ tablespoon sesame oil
$1/4$ tablespoon tamari soy sauce

Dice ginger root. Put all ingredients in blender and blend until smooth.

Pumpkin Seed Dressing

1 cup toasted pumpkin seeds
2 tablespoons brown rice vinegar
1 tablespoon umeboshi vinegar
1 teaspoon tamari soy sauce
1 cup water

Mix in a bowl. Great on cooked greens!

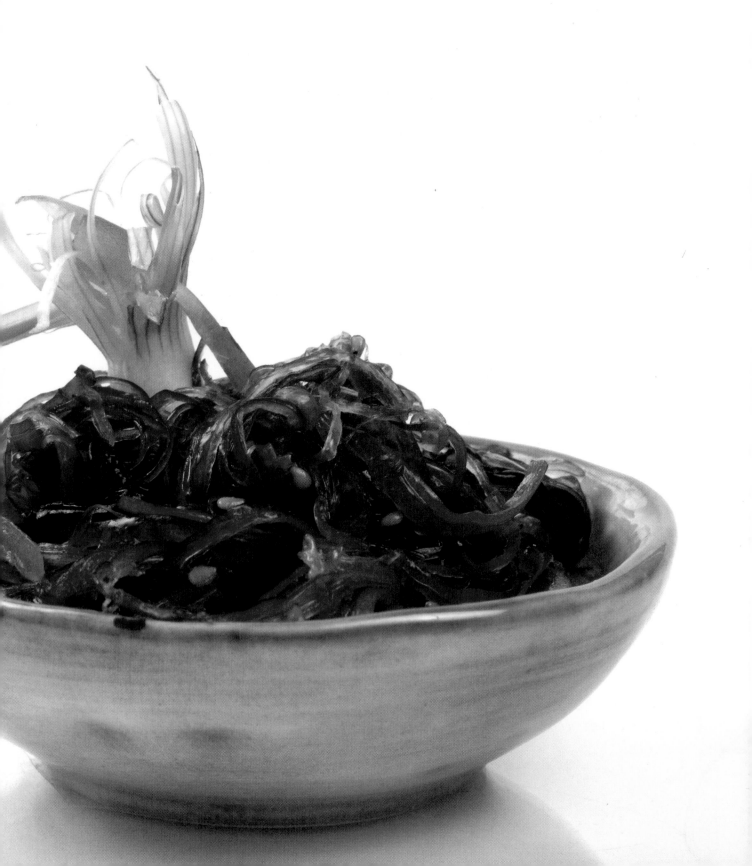

sea vegetables

sea vegetables

Sea vegetables are one of the most nutrition-packed foods on the earth. They are a highly concentrated source of minerals and contain a range of vitamins, all of which nourish you, beautify your skin, hair and nails, and help you feel grounded. They are very versatile, and can be added to soups, salads, stir-fries and desserts. There has been much solid research on the health benefits of sea vegetables; they reduce blood cholesterol, improve digestion, counteract obesity, strengthen bones and teeth, and contain antibiotic properties.

Sea vegetables grown wild and harvested from the ocean are top quality. You can also find high quality brands in your local health food store. Commercially harvested seaweeds are easily found in Asian markets.

So why do so many people wince at the thought of eating seaweed? Maybe it's the thought of fishy taste, slimy texture and funny green color. Below are some recipes for sea vegetables that will help you develop a taste for this wonderful food. Remember, our taste buds often take time to become familiar with new flavors. So give seaweed that "third time is a charm" chance, meaning try one of these seaweeds at least three times, prepared differently each time, before deciding you don't like it.

Arame Mild, semisweet flavor and thin but firm texture. Great as a side dish, but especially yummy with buckwheat.

Hiziki Robust in flavor and black in color. A great side dish.

Kombu Light in flavor and chewy. Expands and softens when soaked. Excellent food tenderizer and helps with the digestibility of beans. Adds a sweet flavor to root vegetables. Creates wonderful stocks and soups.

Nori Paper-thin, dark green sheets made from pressed sea vegetables. Nori has a flavor similar to tuna. Originally used as sushi wrap. Nori flakes may be used as a condiment.

Dulse Savory-tasting, brownish-green-colored stalks. Wonderful for roasting with seeds and as a condiment.

Wakame Delicate, long, green strips. Has a sweet flavor. When soaked, wakame expands a great deal, so cut it into small pieces. Wakame loves the company of carrots and parsnips, and adds a sweet taste to all legumes.

how to clean

Arame and hiziki need to be washed. Although I prefer to soak them as well, some people do not. Soaking will help with their digestability, cooking time and taste.
To soak:

1. Put sea vegetables in a bowl filled with cold water.

2. Move fingers through the stems as if you were shampooing.

3. Discard this "first wash" water.

4. Rinse through again.

5. Fill the bowl with cold water again.

6. Add sea vegetables and let stand for 15 to 20 minutes. Arame requires less time to soak than hiziki.

TIP: Use the water to add to your houseplants or rinse your hair with and watch them grow!

basic cooking for arame and hijiki

After washing and soaking, place them in a pot. Add water and bring to a boil.
Lower heat and simmer for 5 to 10 minutes.

Arame Buckwheat with Onion

½ cup arame
2 cups water
1 cup buckwheat
¼ cup chopped onion

Soak and rinse arame according to directions above.
Bring water to boil.
Slowly add buckwheat, arame and onion.
Cover and simmer on low heat for 20 to 25 minutes.
Do not stir during cooking.

Kung-Fu Hiziki Salad

1 cup hiziki

5 cups water

1 teaspoon sesame oil

2 teaspoons umeboshi vinegar

1 yellow or red pepper

4 stalks scallions

1 carrot

$1/2$ cup corn kernels, fresh off the cob

5 to 6 cherry tomatoes chopped in half (optional)

2 cloves shredded garlic

1 tablespoon fresh ginger juice

Rinse and soak hiziki according to directions above.

Cook hiziki in water for 10 minutes.

Drain from water and allow to cool.

Chop and mix remaining ingredients in a bowl.

Add hiziki.

TIP: *This was Bruce Lee's favorite meal.*

Wakame with Greens

$1/2$ cup wakame, soaked and chopped

1 bunch leafy green vegetables (collards, kale or mustard greens)

1 tablespoon olive oil

Dash of sea salt

Juice of $1/2$ lemon

2 tablespoons gomasio

Wash, soak and chop wakame into small pieces.

Wash and chop greens into bite-size pieces.

Cook wakame in a small amount of water until it becomes tender, about 5 minutes.

In a skillet, heat oil, add greens and sauté for 5 to 7 minutes until leaves wilt.

Add a dash of salt to sauté.

Add soaked wakame and lemon juice.

Sauté together for 3 to 5 more minutes.

Sprinkle with gomasio and serve.

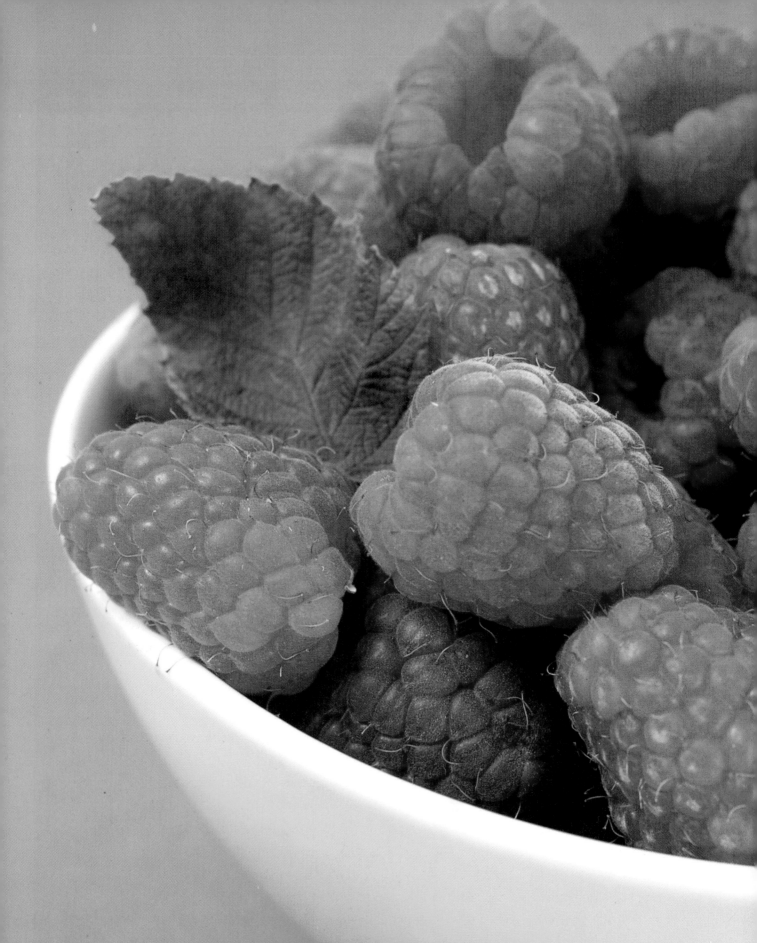

savory snacks

savory snacks

We are a snack foods culture. Grab them on the go. Dip into a treat at that 3:00 to 4:00 pm energy slump. Nibble them while watching a great movie. There are many health-supportive alternatives to processed, quick snack foods. They are tasty, simple and easy to throw in your bag for those days on the go. When those comfort foods and old snack cravings come about, give yourself total permission to enjoy, but try and make these foods at home if possible. Also, check your natural food market for those snacks—like cookies, crackers, chips and sweets—that have higher quality ingredients and more natural substitutes for things such as white flour or sugar than their conventional counterparts.

Here are a few healthy snack ideas:

Various Nuts and Seeds Cashews, peanuts, walnuts, tamari almonds, dry-roasted pumpkin or sunflower seeds.

Trail Mix Create your own custom blend of nuts, seeds and dried fruit from the selection in your local health food store's bulk section.

Baby Carrot Sticks with Hummus A perfect blend of crunchiness and smoothness; make your own hummus or find spiced varieties made without preservatives at your natural food market.

Rice Cakes with Nut Butter We love wild rice cakes with a thin spreading of almond or peanut butter or roasted tahini.

Edamame in a Pod In the frozen food section, a great snack to eat with a sprinkling of sea salt while watching a movie at home.

Fresh Fruit An apple a day… So many different kinds, one day a granny smith the next a gala; or pick from what is in season: pears, plums, peaches, cherries, berries or bananas.

Nori Sheets Found in small on-the-go packs in the seaweed section of your health food store or Asian market, nori is an easy way to get seaweed into your diet.

Granola Homemade or bought in the bulk section, this can be the perfect crunch to keep you going.

Yogurt Whether cow, goat, sheep or soy, we like to buy plain and add our own flavor like sugar-free jam, fresh fruit, granola or a touch of maple syrup.

Mochi A traditional Japanese New Year's treat made from cooked, pureed rice that has been formed into a thick sheet; cut into little cubes and bake for 8 minutes; these little treats are like puff pastries without wheat or flour; found in the refrigerator section of your health food store in savory and sweet flavor, it is a fun snack to have on hand.

Baked Yam Chips Great snack to bring with you when you are on the go. Slice the yam and place on a baking sheet, bake for 20 to 25 minutes at 350 degrees. You can do several at a time to have as snacks throughout the week. They stay good in the fridge for four days.

Ball-O-Nuts

6 dates
$^1/_2$ cup rolled oats
$^3/_4$ cup almonds
$^1/_2$ cup sesame seeds
$^1/_2$ cup apple juice
$^1/_2$ cup brown rice syrup
$^3/_4$ cup poppy seeds

Soak dates with oats in water for a few hours, then drain excess water.
Add all remaining ingredients except poppy seeds into a blender. Blend until chunks become very small, but are still apparent.
Form little balls with the mixture, then roll in poppy seeds.
TIP: You can also squeeze lemon or ginger juice into the mixture.

Kale Chips

1 to 2 bunches kale
Olive oil

Preheat oven to 425 degrees.
Remove kale from stalk, leaving the greens in large pieces.
Place a little olive oil in a bowl, dip your fingers and rub a very light coat of oil over the kale.
Put kale on a baking sheet and bake for 5 minutes or until it starts to turn a bit brown. Keep an eye on it as it can burn quickly. Turn the kale over and bake with the other side up. Remove and serve.
TIP: Try different kinds of kale or collard greens. For added flavor, sprinkle with a little salt or spice such as curry or cumin after rubbing on olive oil.

Parsnip Chips

1 pound parsnips
Olive oil
Sea salt to taste
Black pepper to taste

Preheat oven to 350 degrees.
Wash parsnips well.
Slice parsnips thinly, crosswise, creating circular pieces, and place in a bowl.
Drizzle lightly with olive oil, salt and pepper, and toss so each piece is coated.
Spread evenly over two baking sheets and place in the oven.
Remove after 30 minutes or until desired crispness.

Plantain Chips

6 green plantains
Juice of 6 limes
2 tablespoons coconut oil

To peel the plantains, slice the ends off and cut each plantain in half. Deeply score the skin with a knife, cutting right through to the flesh, down the length of the plantains. Slide your finger under the skin and peel it away.

Slice the plantains diagonally and very thin. Soak the slices in lime juice for 10 to 15 minutes. Then dry thoroughly.

Heat broiler.

Toss plantains with coconut oil in a bowl. Make sure oil covers slices. (You may have to heat the oil just a bit so that it is not in solid form.)

Place on a baking sheet and put under broiler for 3 to 5 minutes or until golden brown.

Flip to the other side, and repeat.

Store refrigerated in an airtight container once cooled down. Keeps for 1 week.

Veggie Muffins

2 cups spelt flour
$1/2$ cup finely chopped fresh parsley
Pinch of sea salt
2 beaten eggs
1 cup grated or finely chopped veggies (whatever you like or have in your fridge)
1 cup soy or rice milk

Preheat oven to 325 degrees.

Mix flour, parsley and salt in a bowl.

Make a well, add eggs and veggies.

Mix lightly, gradually adding milk. This is supposed to be lumpy so don't work too hard!

Scrape into muffin tray that is lightly oiled.

Bake for 12 to15 minutes.

Remove and allow to sit for 10 minutes, then serve.

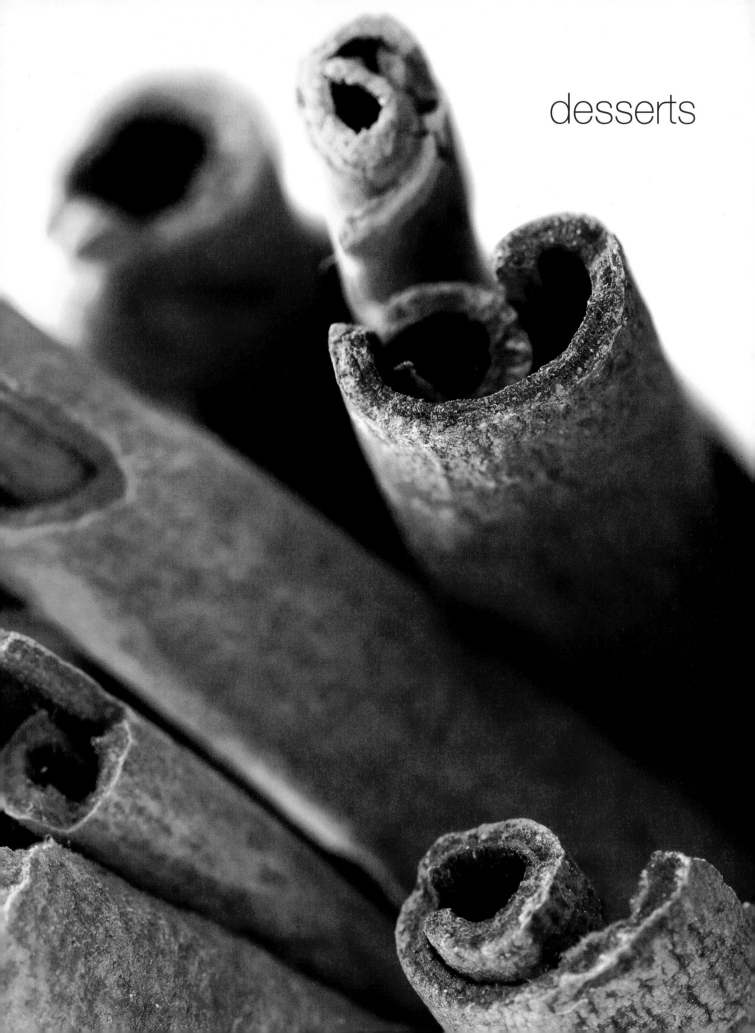

desserts

a good dessert...

...does not take a long time to make

....has all-natural sweet taste, without added
   sugars and chemicals

...can be enjoyed with no guilt and lots of fun

...in small amounts is totally satisfying

...is a chance to be creative in the kitchen

...can act as an invitation for imagination!

Indian Rice Pudding

1 cup white basmati rice

4 cinnamon sticks

1 teaspoon cardamom

2 teaspoons nutmeg

1 teaspoon whole cloves

Shredded lemon peel

Shredded orange peel

2 cups water

$1/2$ cup golden raisins

$1/2$ cup shredded coconut

1 container almond milk

2 tablespoons raw honey

$1/2$ cup pistachios or almonds

Place rice and spices in water and bring to a boil.

Cover and simmer for 20 minutes.

When rice is done, transfer it into a bowl and remove cinnamon sticks.

Mix in raisins and shredded coconut.

Pour almond milk slowly into mixture to achieve your desired consistency.

Add honey and pistachios or almonds.

Baked Bananas

4 firm bananas

1 teaspoon olive oil

1-inch piece grated fresh ginger

1 tablespoon cinnamon

$1/2$ tablespoon nutmeg

$1/2$ cup raisins

Preheat oven to 375 degrees.

Peel and cut bananas in half, lengthwise.

Oil a baking pan and arrange bananas.

Sprinkle with spices and raisins, cover, and bake for 10 to 15 minutes.

TIP: Wonderful with chocolate sauce.

Tofu Ice Cream

18 ounces tofu, well chilled, divided

3 tablespoons honey

$1/4$ tablespoon vanilla extract

$1/8$ teaspoon salt

Combine 12 ounces tofu, honey, vanilla and salt in a blender and puree for about 1 minute.

Transfer to a covered container and place in the freezer overnight.

Next day, cut the frozen tofu into small chunks.

Puree remaining 6 ounces of tofu that is not frozen in the blender until smooth.

While pureeing at high speed, add a few chunks of the frozen tofu at a time into the blender until all has been added and the mixture is smooth and thick.

Serve immediately.

KUZU: THE MAGIC SAUCE THICKENER

You may not know it, but kuzu is very useful in preparing thick sauces, creams and soups. Kuzu is originally from Japan. The white root is made into a powder that dissolves in cold water and becomes thick in hot water. It is all natural, with no bitter or sweet aftertaste. It also has tremendous healing benefits in that it is alkalinizing, soothing, relieves stomach-aches, controls diarrhea, is great for colds and flu, and restores overall strength. Please enjoy experimenting with this amazing powder.

Here is an example of kuzu used in a dessert recipe:

Raisin Pudding

1 cup raisins

2 cups water

1 teaspoon cinnamon

2 tablespoons kuzu

In a saucepan, cook raisins in $1/2$ cup water for 15 minutes.

Add cinnamon if you wish.

When finished cooking, blend in blender.

Meanwhile dissolve kuzu in $1^1/2$ cups water and mix in with blended raisins.

Bring mixture back to saucepan and cook over medium heat for 5 more minutes.

Dash with additional cinnamon and serve.

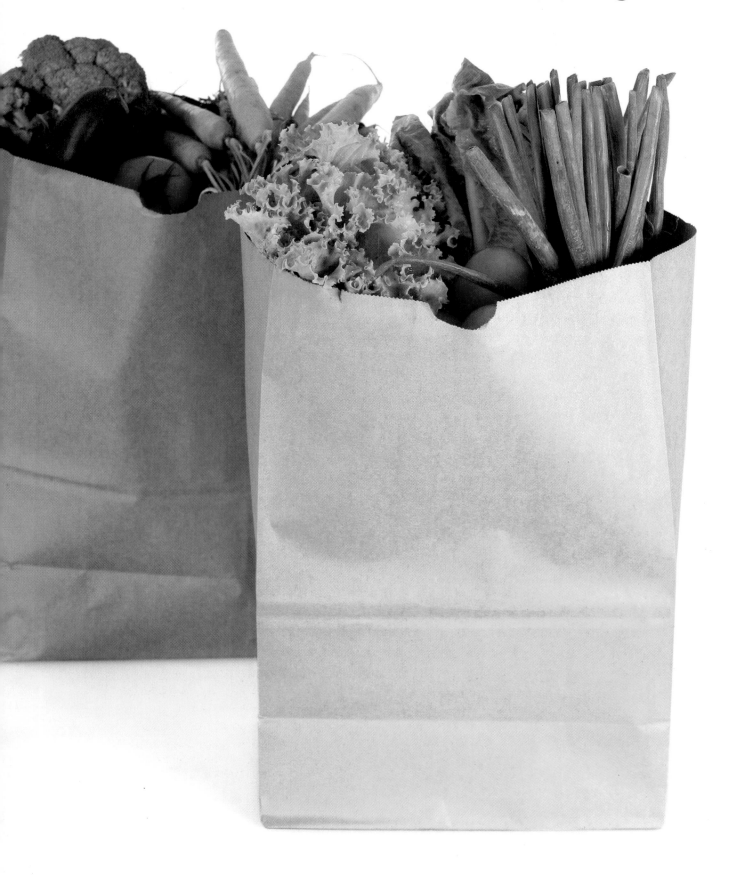

your basic shopping list

your basic shopping list

Many of these items have not been introduced to supermarkets, so you may need to visit your local health food store. Buy organic! It makes a difference! Remember, if you can not find something at the store, you can always find it online.

grains

short grain brown rice

long grain brown rice

white basmati rice

brown basmati rice

millet

barley

rolled oats

buckwheat (also called kasha)

soba noodles

quinoa

beans and soy products

aduki beans

lentils: brown lentils, red lentils, french lentils

garbanzo beans

black beans

split peas

tofu: *fresh soybean curd made of soybean and natural sea salt*

tempeh: *pressed soybean cake made from split soybeans, water and special enzymes*

edamame: *whole, young soybeans in a shell or without; kept frozen*

natto: *whole cooked soybeans fermented with heart-healthy enzymes and whole grains*

sea vegetables

kombu

arame

hijiki

nori: *flakes, whole sheets*

dulse

wakame

condiments

tamari soy sauce

sea salt

umeboshi vinegar: *salty-sour, pickled plum vinegar that originated from Japan; alkalinizing; good salt substitute*

umeboshi plums

balsamic vinegar

natural organic mustard

organic sauerkraut

fresh ginger

fresh garlic

miso (unpasteurized)

bragg's liquid aminos

seeds and nuts

pumpkin seeds

sunflower seeds

poppy seeds

almond, tamari roasted almond

dried chestnut

sesame seeds

spices that are good to have

bay leaf

oregano

thyme

sage

rosemary

dill

fennel

cumin

caraway

mustard seeds

marjoram

garlic

basil

cayenne pepper

butters ORGANIC RECOMMENDED

unsweetened apple butter

toasted sesame seed butter

almond butter

ghee (clarified butter)

sweeteners

brown rice syrup

maple syrup

dried unsulphured fruits: raisins, apricots

raw honey

agave nectar

beverages

kukicha tea/green twig tea

mugicha tea/roasted barley tea

mu tea: *very unique, 16-Chinese-herb-mixture tea*

spring water

peppermint tea

chamomile tea

nettle tea

jasmine tea

dandelion root tea

snacks

baked brown rice crackers: with sesame seeds, seaweed and tamari soy sauce

kamut cakes

toasted seeds

mochi: *a traditional Japanese sweet brown rice cake*

rice syrup candies

amasake: *sweet, velvety-smooth fermented rice beverage; comes in a variety of flavors*

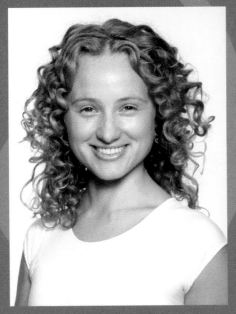

people always ask, "And you are how old?", when I tell them I have my own health and wellness business, the Jena Wellness Group, and manage three employees. "Twenty six," I say, and they are amazed. Only three years after graduating from Integrative Nutrition, the business I created based upon the model taught in the curriculum will gross close to six figures this financial year.

I had two goals when enrolling at the school: to clear up some of my own health concerns and remnants of a teenage eating disorder, and to expand my career. I can happily say that I succeeded in accomplishing both. As the year progressed, the information about a broad spectrum of approaches to food, counseling, and how the body heals fell into place for me. With the support of my personal health counselor, I was able to not only get my own health in order, but also understand how to successfully guide others to do the same. I lost weight, my skin cleared up, cravings diminished, and most profoundly my relationship with food became balanced and healthy after more than 10 years of struggling with it. Feeling healthier gave me more energy to dive into creating my business.

Using Integrative Nutrition's model of the six-month health program as a base, I custom-created my own programs, offering optional massage and private yoga elements, the two healing modalities I had been trained in before going to the school. I applied the marketing strategies taught in the fast-track program, and my clientele steadily grew. Within two years of graduating I had more clients than I could handle, and nine months later made the leap and hired two additional health counselors to see clients and an administrative assistant to help

Jena la Flamme
New York City, NY
Graduate 2002
www.jenawellness.com

run the show. Now I earn money on the days I am not working and can choose to dedicate more of my time to business development, speaking engagements, writing the column I publish in *New York Spirit* magazine and, of course, my personal life.

One of my favorite parts of the freedom of running my own business is that I have been able to take three months of vacation every year. I love traveling! So far in 2005 I have been to Hawaii, Brazil and Bali, places where I can unwind from the task of running a business in New York and be immersed in healing energy.

I can't describe how much my life has changed by going to the school. Being centered in a career that I am interested in and have a gift for, at such a young age, and moreover one that is in a booming industry, is incredible. If this is 26, imagine 36!

epilogue

If you liked this book, you'll love our school. It is a life-changing education within a nurturing environment. We encourage, cultivate and promote good health and nutrition. Our students gain a fundamental and practical knowledge of traditional and modern approaches to nutrition, of East and West, and, most importantly, a profound understanding of themselves.

We at Integrative Nutrition believe that our graduates are the counselors best prepared to help clients achieve a lifetime of good health and empowerment.

The Institute for Integrative Nutrition is located at:
3 East 28th Street, Floor 12
New York City, NY 10016

www.integrativenutrition.com
212.730.5433

references

The 3-Season Diet: Eat the Way Nature Intended: Lose Weight, Beat Food Cravings, Get Fit by John Douillard, PhD. Three Rivers Press, 2000.

The Art of Listening by Harvey Jackins. Rational Island Publishers, 1981.

Can't Buy My Love: How Advertising Changes the Way We Think and Feel by Jean Kilbourne. Touchstone, 1999.

*Diet for a Small Plan*et by Frances Moore Lappé. Ballantine Books, 1972.

Eat, Drink and Be Healthy: The Harvard Medical School Guide to Healthy Eating by Walter Willett, MD. Free Press, 2001.

Eat More, Weigh Less by Dean Ornish, MD. HarperCollins Publishers, 1993.

Eat Right for Your Type: The Individualized Diet Solution to Staying Healthy, Living Healthy & Achieving Your Ideal Weight by Peter D'Adamo, ND. GP Putnam's Sons, 1996.

Energetics of Food: Encounters with Your Most Intimate Relationship by Steve Gagné. Spiral Sciences, 1990.

Enter the Zone: The Dietary Road Map to Lose Weight & More by Barry Sears, PhD and Bill Lawren. HarperCollins Publishers, 1995.

The Five Phases of Food: How to Begin by John Garvy, Jr., ND, DAc. Well Being Books, 1985.

Food and Our Bones: The Natural Way to Prevent Osteoporosis by Annemarie Colbin, PhD. The Penguin Group, 1998.

Food Politics: How the Food Industry Influences Nutrition and Health by Marion Nestle, PhD, MPH. University of California Press, 2002.

Get the Sugar Out: 501 Simple Ways to Cut the Sugar out of Any Diet by Ann Louise Gittleman, PhD, CNS. Three Rivers Press, 1996.

The Glucose Revolution Life Plan by Jennie Brand-Miller, Avalon Publishing Group, 2001.

Healing with Whole Foods: Asian Traditions and Modern Nutrition by Paul Pitchford. North Atlantic Books, 1993.

The Master Cleanser: With Special Needs and Problems by Stanley Burroughs. Burroughs Books, 1976.

Nature's First Law: The Raw-Food Diet by Stephen Arllin, Fouad Dini and David Wolfe. Maul Brothers Publishing, 1996.

Nourishing Traditions: The Cookbook That Challenges Politically Correct Nutrition and the Diet Dictocrats by Sally Fallon with Mary Enig, PhD. NewTrends Publishing, 1999.

Nourishing Wisdom: A Mind-Body Approach to Nutrition and Well-Being by Marc David, with Patrick McGrady, Jr. Bell Tower, 1991.

Power Eating Program: You Are How You Eat by Lino Stanchich. Healthy Products, Inc., 1989.

Pritikin Program for Diet and Exercise by Nathan Pritikin, MD. Grosset and Dunlap, 1980.

The Self-Healing Cookbook: A Macrobiotic Primer for Healing Body, Mind and Moods with Whole, Natural Foods by Kristina Turner. Earthtones Press, 1987.

Soul Work: Finding the Work You Love, Loving the Work You Find by Deborah Bloch and Lee Richmond. Davies-Black Publishing, 1998.

The South Beach Diet: The Delicious, Doctor Designed, Foolproof Plan for Fast and Healthy Weight Loss by Arthur Agatston, MD. Rodale, Inc, 2003.

Staying Healthy with the Seasons by Elson M. Haas, MD. Celestial Arts, 1981.

The Truth about Drug Companies: How They Deceive Us and What to Do about It by Marcia Angell, MD. Random House Publishing Group, 2004.

Your Body's Many Cries For Water: You Are Not Sick, You Are Thirsty! by Fereydoon Batmanghelidj, MD. Global Health Solutions, 1992.

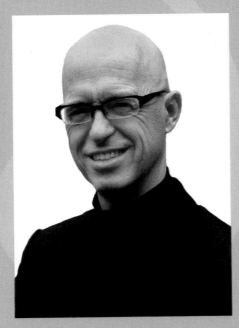

the author

JOSHUA ROSENTHAL IS FOUNDER, director and primary teacher of the Institute for Integrative Nutrition in New York City. He is a trained therapist with a Masters of Science in Education, specializing in counseling. With over 25 years' experience in the fields of whole foods, personal coaching, curriculum development, teaching and nutritional counseling, he is a highly sensitive healer whose enthusiasm shines through in all his work. His simple approach allows people to quickly and successfully reach new levels of health and happiness.

index

a

aduki beans
    Basic, 179
    Squash Stew, 179
advertising, 22, 97, 98
Agatston, Arthur, 52
agave nectar, 69, 127–28
allergies, 8, 44
    to dairy, 129
    to soy, 117
    to wheat, 9, 48, 114
American Dietetic Association
    (ADA), 13–14
American Medical Association
    (AMA), 48
ancestry, 21, 43, 130
Angell, Marcia, 12
antibiotics, 7, 50, 117, 129, 130
arame, 201, 202
    Buckwheat with Carrot and, 166
Arugula and Beef Stir-Fry, 188
Atkins, Robert, 49–50, 51, 52
authentic self-expression, 152–53
awareness exercises, 89
Ayurveda, 43–46, 75

b

Bananas, Baked, 210
barley malt, 128
Batmanghelidj, Fereydoon, 28
beans, 24, 53, 117, 126
    recipes for, 177–81, 195
    shopping list for, 213
beef, 11, 24, 68, 68, 71, 117
    antibiotics in, 7, 50, 130
    recipes for, 188
beer, 52, 70
Beet-Carrot-Parsnip-Fennel
    Extravaganza, 174
being bad, 134
beverages, shopping list for, 213
binging, 27
bio-individuality, 21–22
    protein requirements and, 116

bitter foods, 70
blood sugar, 49, 52, 64–65, 72,
    126–27
    stevia and, 128
    whole grains and, 114
    Zone diet and, 51
blood type, 53–54, 116, 130
body
    as laboratory, 22, 30, 40
    listening to, 22–23, 27, 31, 32–33,
    42, 57
    loving relationship with, 73
    writing a letter to, 76
Bok Choy Stir-Fry, 172
bone fractures and osteoporosis, 8,
    53, 129
Brand-Miller, Jennie, 52
bread, 5, 9, 47, 51, 66
breakfast, 32–33, 64, 111, 143
broccoli
    Garlic Gingered, with Toasted
    Pumpkin Seeds, 172
    Soup, Creamy, 193
brown rice syrup, 64, 69, 127
buckwheat, 113
    with Carrot and Arame, 166
    Very Russian, 166
burdock
    Carrot Power Meal, 175
    Millet-Carrot-Hiziki, 167
Burroughs, Stanley, 55
butters, 213

c

Cabbage, Sautéed, 173
caffeine, 95, 131
    coffee, 28–29, 68, 70, 100, 118,
    131
calcium, 129
calories, 25–27
cancer, 7, 25, 50, 53, 54, 71, 81,
    116,130
    breast, 8, 53, 129
candida, 48, 49, 114

carbohydrates, 6
    chewing of, 31
    in Fallon diet, 54
    in food pyramid, 5, 6
    high carbohydrate diets, 47–48,
    113
    high protein diets and, 49, 50
    metabolic rate and, 26
    overweight associated with, 64,
    113
    simple and complex, 63–65, 126
    in South Beach diet, 52
    in Zone diet, 51
career, 86–87, 119, 153
carrot(s), 205
    -Beet-Parsnip-Fennel
    Extravaganza, 174
    Buckwheat with Arame and, 166
    Burdock Power Meal, 175
    Ginger Soup, 192
    -Millet-Hiziki-Burdock, 167
Celery Root, Roasted Rutabaga with,
    174
cereals, 5, 9
cheese, 52, 68, 71, 129
chewing, 30–31, 34, 71
chicken, 7, 24, 68, 117, 130
    recipes for, 189, 193
chickpeas
    Basic, 180
    Hummus, 181
    Veggie Bake, 175
children, 66, 97, 126
Chili, Vegetarian Bean, 181
China
    5 Element Theory in, 46–47
    medicine in, 4, 13, 70
chocolate, 56, 68, 69–70, 132
circle of life exercise, 90
Cod Fish, Ideal Dill, 187
coffee, 28–29, 68, 70, 100, 118, 131
Collards with Dill and Parsley, 174
communication, 84, 85–86
community, 83

condiments, 143, 146, 213

cooking, 111–13, 139–46

    salt in, 131–32

    seasonal, 143–44

    simplicity in, 142–43

    see also recipes

corn syrup, 11

cravings, 27, 41, 48, 57, 63–73, 113

    inventory of, 74

    protein and, 116

    for sugar and sweets, 55, 63–64,
        65, 69–70, 110, 114, 116

    tongue scraper and, 75, 118

    for water, 110, 111

cross-species transference, 24, 130

crowding out, 28–29, 57, 131

d

D'Adamo, James, 53

D'Adamo, Peter, 53, 130

Daikon Radish, Steamed, with Black
    Sesame Seeds, 173

dairy industry, 5, 8, 47

dairy products, 6, 24, 48, 67, 71, 117,
    118, 128–30

    blood type and, 53

    as contracting food, 68

    fats in, 54, 129

    raw, 54

    tongue scraper and, 75

    USDA recommendations for, 5, 8

date sugar, 128

David, Marc, 62

dehydration, see water

depression, 82

desserts, 209–11

diabetes, 6, 7, 49, 52, 72, 81, 126

diet(s)

    Atkins, 49–50, 51, 52

    Ayurveda and, 43–46

    binging and, 27

    bio-individuality and, 21–22, 116

    blood type and, 53–54, 116, 130

    creating your own, 58

    finding the right one for you, 57

    5 Element Theory, 46–47

    high carbohydrate, 47–48

    high protein, 49–50, 52, 64, 65

    Joshua's 90–10, 57

    lemonade, 55–56

macrobiotic, 39–40, 42–43, 48

metabolism and, 26–27

raw food, 55

Sally Fallon, 54

South Beach, 52

truth in, 41

Zone, 50–51

    see also eating; food

Dietary Goals for the U.S., 6

Dietary Guidelines, 7–9, 22

Diet for a Small Planet (Lappé), 47

digestion, 27, 29–30, 31, 53, 71

    bitter foods and, 70

    exercise and, 119

disease and illness, 3, 6, 7, 8, 25, 81

    animal food and, 116

    cooked food and, 55

    Master Cleanser and, 55

    protein and, 53

    water intake and, 28

doctors, 3–5, 12–13

drug companies, 4, 11, 12–13

drugs, 3, 4, 28, 95

dulse, 201

e

Eat, Drink and Be Healthy (Willett), 8

eating

    contemporary habits of, 7

    environment and, 30, 31

    overeating, 27

    seasonal, 29, 42, 44, 46, 47, 55,
        143–44

    slowly, 31, 34

    time of day and, 29–30

    see also diet; food

Eat More, Weigh Less (Ornish), 47–48

Eat Right for Your Type (D'Adamo), 53

Edison, Thomas, 2

eggs, 6, 24, 52, 54, 68, 117

elements, five, 44, 46–47

*Energetics of Food: Encounters with
    Your Most Intimate Relationship*
    (Gagné), 23–24

energy, 23–25, 30, 70

    cooking and, 140

    metabolic rate and, 25–27

    overeating and, 27

    water and, 110, 111

enzymes, 55, 70, 116, 126

exercise, 46, 47, 87, 119

    craving for, 72

    metabolic rate and, 26

    USDA and, 7, 8, 9–11

exercises

    being bad, 134

    breakfast, 32–33

    circle of life, 90

    condiment list, 146

    craving inventory, 74

    creating your own diet, 58

    first step in Integrative Nutrition
        plan, 120

    future-building, 154–56

    hot towel scrub, 118, 120

    hot water bottle, 104, 118

    metabolic type, 34

    mindful eating, 34

    MyPyramid, 15

    reducing one food, 133

    supermarket field trip, 15

    Supersize Me, 16

    tongue scraper, 75, 118

    trustworthy professionals, 16

    trying a new recipe, 146

    turning off the media, 102

    wish list, 103

    writing a letter to your
        body, 76

f

Fallon, Sally, 54, 114

family, 118

farmers, 11

fasting, 56, 57

fats and oils, 7, 48, 70, 71, 116

    in Atkins diet, 49, 50

    in chocolate, 132

    in dairy products, 54, 129

    in Fallon diet, 54

    in food pyramid, 5

    hydrogenated, 8, 11

    in South Beach diet, 52

    trans, 8, 48, 50, 71, 132

    in Zone diet, 51

FDA (Food and Drug Administration),
    4, 12

Fennel-Beet-Carrot-Parsnip
    Extravaganza, 174

fiber, 64, 65, 66

fish, 24, 47, 68, 71–72, 117
    recipes for, 187
fitting in and fitting out, 100–101,
    151–52
5 Element Theory, 46–47
flexitarians, 145
food(s)
    to avoid or minimize, 125–34
    chewing of, 30–31, 34, 71
    contracting and expanding, 68–69
    cravings for, see cravings
    cross-species transference and,
        24, 130
    crowding out, 28–29, 57, 131
    cutting out one from your diet,
        56–57
    energy of, 23–25
    extreme, 68–69, 70, 153
    fast, 6, 7, 8, 11, 12, 13, 22, 41, 95,
        100, 131, 141
    freshness of, 140–41
    instant gratification and, 96–97
    junk, 8, 11, 22, 29, 55, 66, 68, 69,
        95, 97, 113, 118, 131, 152
    locally grown, 29, 42, 44, 140–41,
        143
    organic, 25, 50, 117, 129, 130,
        131, 132
    politics of, 6, 8, 11, 13
    primary, see primary foods
    processed and refined, 6, 7, 9, 25,
        55, 64, 65, 66, 68, 69, 70, 117
    quality of, 25
    raw, 55, 71
    secondary, 81, 82, 89
    see also diet; eating
food industry, 6, 8, 11, 13, 14
food journals, 23, 47, 74
Food Politics: How the Food Industry
    Influences Nutrition and Health
        (Nestle), 5
food pyramids
    Atkins, 50
    Integrative Nutrition, 89
    USDA, 4, 5, 6, 9–11, 15, 22, 24
freedom, 96
friendships, 82–83, 118, 145
fruits, 11, 24, 47, 55, 64, 71, 126, 205
    in food pyramid, 5
    organic, 25

seasonal eating and, 29, 44, 143
    in Zone diet, 51
future, 152–53, 154–56

g
Gagné, Steve, 23–24
Gandhi, Mahatma, 20
garlic
    Gingered Broccoli with Toasted
        Pumpkin Seeds, 172
    Ginger Parsley Dressing, 199
    Steamed String Beans, 171
ginger, 70
    Carrot Soup, 192
    Chicken Soup, 193
    Garlic Broccoli with Toasted
        Pumpkin Seeds, 172
    Parsley Garlic Dressing, 199
Gittleman, Anne Louise, 48
gluten, 48, 114
glycemic index, 52
government, 3, 6, 8, 11–12, 98
    FDA, 4, 12
    USDA, 4, 5, 6, 7–11
grains, 47, 51, 64, 126
    Ayurveda and, 44
    blood type and, 53
    gluten in, 48, 114
    macrobiotics and, 42
    phytic acid in, 54, 114
    preparation and recipes for,
        113–14, 143, 162–67, 195
    shopping list for, 213
    water content of, 111
    whole, 7, 8–9, 11, 47, 48, 54, 64,
        65, 66, 113–14, 126, 129
greens, 11, 24, 33, 65, 70, 115–16,
    129
    Sautéed, in Olive Oil, 171
    Steamed Kale, 171
    Wakame with, 203

h
Healing with Whole Foods: Asian
    Traditions and Modern Nutrition
        (Pitchford), 43
health, 151–53
healthcare system, 3–5, 12–13
heart disease, 6, 7, 48, 50, 53, 54,
    71–72, 81, 116, 117, 129, 130

high blood pressure, 81, 116, 117,
    131
Hippocrates, 160
hiziki, 201, 202
    Kung-Fu Salad, 203
    Millet-Carrot-Burdock, 167
honey, 128
hormones, 50, 117, 129, 130
hot towel scrub, 118, 120
hot water bottle, 104, 118
hummus, 205
    recipe for, 181
hunger, 27, 48
hypoglycemia, 72, 126

i
ice cream, 57, 66–67, 71, 129
Ice Cream, Tofu, 211
illness, see disease and illness
India, 29
    Ayurveda system of, 43–46, 75
individuality, 21–22
    protein requirements and, 116
instincts, 22, 27, 67–68
Institute for Integrative Nutrition, ix, 5,
    40, 41, 100, 217
    ADA and, 14
    Food Pyramid of, 89
    graduate profiles, 17, 35, 59, 77,
        91, 105, 121, 135, 147, 157, 215
Integrative Nutrition plan, 109–20
intimacy, 83, 84

j
Jamieson, Alex, 12
Japanese diet, 6, 21, 113, 117
    macrobiotic, 39–40, 42–43, 48
journals, food, 23, 47, 74
Jung, Carl, 88

k
kale
    Chips, 206
    Steamed, 171
Kalish, Julia, 59
kapha principle, 44, 45
Kennedy, Teresa Kay-Aba, 35
kombu, 201
Kushi, Michio and Avalene, 39–40
kuzu, 211

la Flamme, Jena, 215
Lao Tzu, 108
Lappé, Frances Moore, 47
Leek Meatballs, Spicy, 188
leftovers, 140, 143
Lemonade Diet, 55–56
Lemon Tahini Dressing, 199
lentil
French, Shiitake Salad, 196
Minty Green, Watercress Salad, 197
Red, Burgers, 180
listening, 22–23
to your body, 22–23, 27, 31, 32–33, 42, 57
love, 81, 82, 83, 84
in food, 141
lovemaking, 84–85
lunch, 64–65, 143

m

McDonald's, 8, 11, 12
McDougall, John, 47
McGovern, George, 47
macrobiotics, 39–40, 42–43, 48
maple syrup, 128
marriage, 101, 118
massage, 84, 85
Master Cleanser, 55–56
matrix, 95–101, 151
meat, 6, 25, 33, 44, 47, 95, 100, 116–18, 130–31
in Atkins diet, 49, 50, 52
blood type and, 53, 116, 130
as contracting food, 68
cravings for, 41, 68
in Fallon diet, 54
in food pyramid, 5, 24
hormones and antibiotics in, 7, 50, 130
organic, 117
recipes for, 188
in South Beach diet, 52
meat industry, 5, 6, 8, 47
media, 98
turning off, 102
medical system, 3–5, 12–13
medicines, 3, 4, 28, 95
drug companies and, 4, 11, 12–13

men, superman syndrome and, 99–100
metabolism, 25–27, 34
milk, 9, 53, 54, 71, 128
organic, 129
see also dairy products
millet, 113
-Carrot-Hiziki-Burdock, 167
with Roasted Sunflower Seeds, 166
Winter Squash and, 167
minerals, 48, 65, 66, 126
phytic acid and, 114
in salt, 70, 132
miso, 42, 43, 48, 117
Soup, Mighty, 191
Soup, Shiitake, 191
mochi, 205
models, 98
molasses, 128
moods, 23
Morning Glory with Oats, 163
Muesli, 163
Muffins, Veggie, 207
Murray, W. H., x
mushrooms
French Lentil Shiitake Salad, 196
Shiitake Miso Soup, 191
MyPyramid, 9–11, 15, 22

n

nervous systems, 26, 30
Nestle, Marion, 5, 6
nori, 201, 205
Northrup, Christiane, 38, 39
Notter, Robert, 77
Nourishing Traditions: The Cookbook That Challenges Politically Correct Nutrition and the Diet Dictocrats (Fallon), 54
nuts, 24, 44, 52, 205, 213
Ball-O-Nuts, 206

o

oats, 113
Morning Glory with, 163
Muesli, 163
Ohsawa, George, 39, 42
Ohsawa, Lima, 124
organic food, 25, 50, 117, 129, 130,

131, 132
Ornish, Dean, 39, 47–48
osho, 80
osteoporosis, 8, 53, 129
overweight and obesity, 3, 6, 6, 7, 8, 11, 12, 81, 116
carbohydrates associated with, 64, 113

p

parsnip
-Beet-Carrot-Fennel Extravagaza, 174
Chips, 206
parties, 143, 144
pasta, 5, 47, 51
Patton, Diana, 147
Payne, Rose, 91
Pea, Split, Soup, 192–93
pesticides, 25
physical activity, 87, 119
see also exercise
phytic acid, 54, 114
phytochemicals, 66
Pitchford, Paul, 39, 43
pitta principle, 44, 45
placebo effect, 41
Plantain Chips, 207
politics, 6, 8, 11, 13
Popper, Pamela, 14
pork, 11, 68
potato chips, 6, 11, 48, 71
poultry, 24, 47
chicken, 7, 24, 68, 117, 130, 193
recipes for, 188, 189, 193
Power Eating Program: You Are How You Eat (Stanchich), 30
Price, Weston, 54
primary foods, 81–90
career, 86–87, 119, 153
cooking and, 140
physical activity, 87, 119
relationships, 82–86, 118, 145, 153
spirituality, 88–89, 119, 153
Pritikin, Nathan, 47
Pritikin Longevity Center, 47, 48
protein, 68, 70, 131
in Atkins diet, 49, 50, 52
blood type and, 53, 116

experimenting with, 116–18

in food pyramids, 5, 9, 24

high protein diets, 49–50, 52, 64, 65

metabolic rate and, 26

in milk, 54

in raw food diet, 55

in South Beach diet, 52

in vegetarian diet, 54, 117

in Zone diet, 50–51

pumpkin seed(s), 205

Dressing, 199

Toasted, Garlic Gingered Broccoli with, 172

pungent flavors, 70

q

quinoa, 113

Salad, 195

Spring Out, 167

r

Raisin Pudding, 211

raw foods, 55, 71

recipes, 142, 146, 162–211

beans, 177–81, 195

desserts, 209–11

grains, 113–14, 162–67, 195

meat and fish, 187–89

salad dressings, 199

salads, 165, 195–98

sea vegetables, 201–3

shopping list for, 213

snacks, 205–7

soups, 191–93

tofu and tempeh, 183–85, 211

vegetables, 115, 169–75

relationships, 82–86, 118, 145, 153

religion, 88, 119

restaurants, 131, 144–45

cost and, 142

fast food, 6, 7, 8, 11, 12, 13, 22, 41, 95, 100, 131, 141

rice, 5, 24, 42

Basic Brown, Pot, 163

Brown, Sesame Dulse, 164

Golden, 164

Indian Pudding, 210

preparation of, 112, 113–14

Salad, Gypsies' Singing, 165

Very Easy Fried, 165

Wild, 164

rice cakes, 64, 69, 71, 205

rice syrup, 64, 69, 127

Rosenbloom, Steve, 135

Rossetto, Devon, 17

Rutabaga, Roasted, with Celery Root, 174

s

salad dressing recipes, 199

salads, 71, 112, 116

recipes for, 165, 195–98

seasonal eating and, 29

Salmon Cake, 187

salt, 131–32

as contracting food, 68

craving for, 70

in Japanese diet, 42, 43

Sarfati, Debbie, 157

Sears, Barry, 50–51, 117

seasonal affective disorder, 144

seasonal eating, 29, 42, 44, 46, 47, 55, 143–44

sea vegetables, 48, 70

calcium in, 129

recipes for, 201–3

shopping list for, 213

seeds, 205, 213

see also pumpkin seed; sesame seed; sunflower seeds

self-expression, 152–53

sensuality and sexuality, 84–85

sesame seed(s)

Dulse Brown Rice, 164

Element Dressing, 199

Steamed Daikon Radish with, 173

Shaw, George Bernard, 150

shopping list, 213

snacks, 29, 72, 143, 205

recipes for, 205–7

shopping list for, 213

Snickers, 96–97

soba noodles, 70

Cold, Salad, 198

soft drinks, 8, 11, 13, 28, 114

soups, 29, 111, 143

recipes for, 191–93

South Beach diet, 52

soy beans and soy products, 11, 42, 117

shopping list for, 213

tofu and tempeh, 117, 183–85, 211

Soy Zone, 4

spices, shopping list for, 213

spicy foods, 70–71

spirituality, 27, 88–89, 119, 153

Splenda, 127

Spurlock, Morgan, 12, 16

squash, winter

Aduki Stew, 179

and Millet, 167

Stanchich, Lino, 30–31

stevia, 128

subsidization, 11

sucralose, 127

sugar and sweets, 11, 14, 55, 56, 64–65, 66, 68, 72, 95, 118, 125–28

alternatives to, 69, 127–28, 213

Atkins diet and, 49, 50

blood sugar and, see blood sugar

in chocolate, 132

cravings for, 55, 63–64, 65, 69–70, 110, 114, 116

Dietary Guidelines and, 7, 8

as expanding food, 68

in food pyramid, 5

hypoglycemia and, 72, 126

sunflower seeds, 205

Roasted, Millet with, 166

superman syndrome, 99–100

supermarket field trip, 15

Supersize Me, 12, 16

superwoman syndrome, 99

supportive relationships, 118

Sweet Potato with Rosemary, Baked Caraway, 175

Sweet Sensation, 115

synchronicity, 88–89

t

tahini

Hummus, 181

Lemon Dressing, 199

tea, 28, 66, 111, 131, 213

tempeh, 183

recipes for, 185

Terjesen, Donna, 121

Thompson, Tommy, 7
tofu, 117, 183
    recipes for, 183, 184, 211
tongue scraper, 75, 118
touch, hugs and cuddles, 84, 85
toxins, 56
trustworthy professionals, 16
Truth About Drug Companies, The:
    How They Deceive Us and What
    to Do About It (Angell), 12

U

USDA (U.S. Department of Agriculture)
    Dietary Guidelines, 7–9, 22
    Food Guide Pyramid, 4, 5, 6
    MyPyramid, 9–11, 15, 22
U.S. Department of Health and
    Human Services, 5, 7
U.S. Senate Select Committee on
    Nutrition and Human Needs, 6, 8, 47
U.S. Surgeon General, 48

V

vata principle, 44
vegans, 116–17, 130
vegetables, 7, 11, 29, 56, 64, 65, 66,
    70, 72, 113, 126
    blood type and, 53
    calcium in, 129

energy of, 24
in food pyramids, 5, 9, 11
green leafy, see greens
in high carbohydrate diets, 47, 48
organic, 25
preparation of, 112, 116, 143
recipes for, 115, 169–75
sea, see sea vegetables
seasonal eating and, 29, 44, 143
in South Beach diet, 52
sweet, 65, 69, 114–15
water content of, 111
in Zone diet, 51
vegetarianism, 41, 49, 118, 130
    blood type and, 53
    protein needs and, 54, 117
    seasonal eating and, 29
    Zone diet and, 51
Veggie Muffins, 207
vitamins, 65, 66, 70
Vitti, Alisa, 105

W

wakame, 201
    with Greens, 203
water, 11, 28–29, 33, 66, 71, 110–11, 131
    hot, with lemon, 111
    macrobiotic diet and, 43
    Zone diet and, 51

Watercress Lentil Salad, Minty Green,
    197
weight loss, 48, 65
    high protein diets and, 49, 50
    South Beach diet and, 52
wheat, 11, 53, 114
    allergies to, 9, 48, 114
    gluten in, 48, 114
Willett, Walter, 8, 129
willpower and discipline, 41, 63,
    67–68
wish list, 103
Woolf, Virginia, 138
women
    and pressure to be thin, 97–98
    and superwoman syndrome, 99
work, 86–87, 119, 153

Y

yam chips, 205
yin-yang philosophy, 42, 48, 55, 110
yogurt, 67, 117, 205
Your Body's Many Cries for Water
    (Batmanghelidj), 28

Z

Zen Buddhism, 100
Zohar, Zemach, 94
Zone diet, 50–51, 117